T0241864

Small Incision Lenticule Extraction (SMILE)

Walter Sekundo

Editor

Small Incision Lenticule Extraction (SMILE)

Principles, Techniques, Complication Management, and Future Concepts

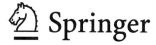 Springer

Editor
Walter Sekundo
Department of Ophthalmology
Philipps University of Marburg
and
Universitätsklinikum Giessen & Marburg GmbH
Marburg
Germany

ISBN 978-3-319-37226-6   ISBN 978-3-319-18530-9   (eBook)
DOI 10.1007/978-3-319-18530-9

Springer Cham Heidelberg New York Dordrecht London
© Springer International Publishing Switzerland 2015
Softcover reprint of the hardcover 1st edition 2015

Springer International Publishing AG Switzerland is part of Springer Science+Business Media
(www.springer.com)

Contents

Author Biographies

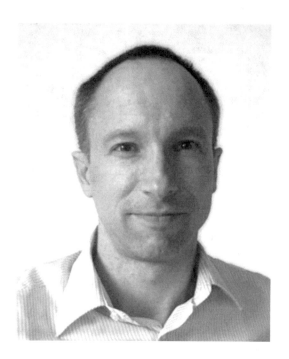

Mark Bischoff is Director, Research and Development for Refractive Lasers, at Carl Zeiss Meditec AG. He joined ZEISS in 2002, where he has worked on the development project for the femtosecond laser system VisuMax and the SMILE procedure. In 2004, he became manager of this project and in 2006 head of the systems engineering team. Since 2008, he has been the director of R&D for refractive lasers. Mark Bischoff received his doctorate in physics in 2000 from the Friedrich Schiller University Jena. He then joined the manufacturer of femtosecond fiber lasers, IMRA America, Inc. in Ann Arbor, MI (USA), before he went to the University of Jena as postdoc and leader of an industry project.

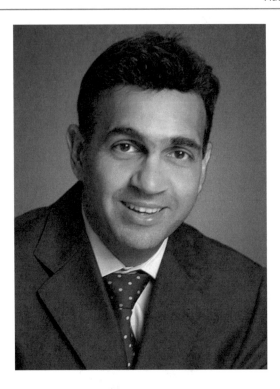

Jodhbir S. Mehta is Head of the Tissue Engineering and Stem Cell Group at the Singapore Eye Research Institute and Head of the Corneal Service and Senior Consultant in the Refractive Service of the Singapore National Eye Center (SNEC). He has academic affiliations with DUKE-NUS GMS.

He has won 25 national and international awards including those at AAO and ARVO. His interests lie in corneal transplantation—penetrating keratoplasty, lamellar keratoplasty, endothelial keratoplasty, femtosecond laser technology, corneal imaging, corneal infections, corneal refractive surgery, keratoprosthesis surgery, ocular drug delivery systems, and corneal genetics. He has authored over 210 peer-reviewed publications and 9 book chapters and given over 210 oral and poster presentations. His research work has developed nine patents, two of which have been commercialized and licensed to companies.

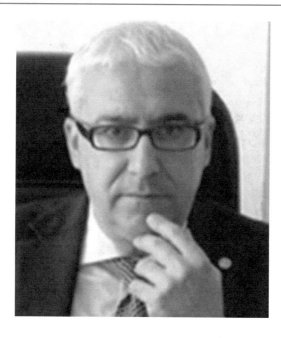

Leonardo Mastropasqua is Full Professor, Diseases of the Visual System, Faculty of Medicine and Surgery, "G. d'Annunzio" University of Chieti-Pescara. Currently, he is Head of the National High-Technology Center in Ophthalmology and the Center of Excellence in Ophthalmology, National President of the Ophthalmology Society of Italian Universities (SOU), President of the Italian Council of University Professors of Ophthalmology, Scientific Advisor of the Directive Council of the Italian section of IAPB (International Agency for the Prevention of Blindness), and Board Member of the EUCORNEA Society.

He has authored over 240 original scientific articles, book chapters, and monographs in ophthalmology, 125 of which are published in peer-reviewed journals included in the *Journal Citation Reports*.

His principal fields of interest include refractive surgery, corneal pathologies and surgery, cataract surgery, glaucoma, and advanced ophthalmic imaging. He does more than 4,000 surgical procedures per year (anterior and posterior segment) and approximately 2,000 refractive procedures.

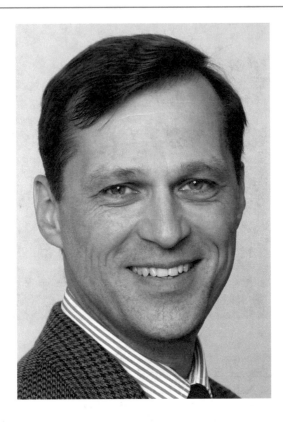

Marcus Blum was born 1 August 1960 in Kassel and grew up in Karlsruhe, Germany. After military service, he started his medical education at the University of Heidelberg and was trained in the Department of Ophthalmology at Heidelberg (by Prof. H.E. Völcker). In 1994, he took the board exam and moved to Jena as a fellow (under Prof. J. Strobel). He was appointed Associate Professor at the University of Jena in 1999. Dr. Blum was involved in building up a technology network focusing on new technologies for ophthalmology in Jena. In 2001, he became head of the Ophthalmology Department at the HELIOS Klinikum Erfurt. He is clinical investigator for Carl Zeiss Meditec.

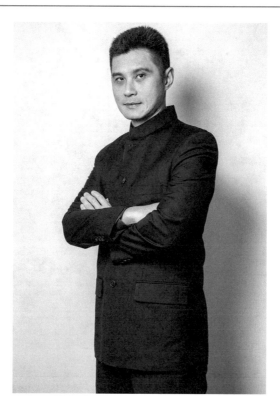

Ekktet Chansue, MD is the Medical Director of TRSC International LASIK Center in Bangkok, Thailand. After finishing his Cornea, External Disease and Refractive Surgery fellowship in St. Louis, MO, in 1993, he taught at the Ramathibodi Hospital Faculty of Medicine, Mahidol University, Bangkok, for several years. Dr. Chansue performed the first LASIK in Thailand (and probably in South East Asia) in 1994 and has since performed more than 30,000 LASIKs. Dr. Chansue also performed the first ReLEx® SMILE in Thailand in 2010. He designed the Chansue ReLEx® Dissector, an instrument to aid in the separation and freeing of the lenticule during the ReLEx® procedure.

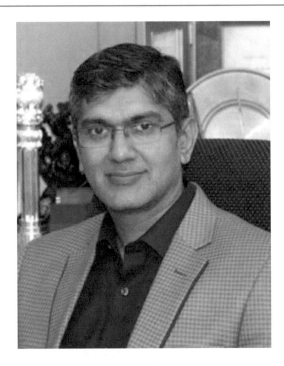

Sri Ganesh is Chairman and Managing Director, Nethradhama Hospital Pvt. Ltd, Bangalore

He received his basic medical education from Bangalore University and completed his postgraduate training at Regional Institute of Ophthalmology, Bangalore. He did observership in Phacoemulsification and Lasik at Sheppard Eye Centre, LV, Nevada, USA.

He is recognized for his expertise in cataract and refractive surgery and has performed over 50 live surgeries at various national and international conferences. He has a special interest in latest technology such as the femtosecond laser-assisted cataract surgery and all femtosecond laser refractive correction (ReLEx SMILE).

He was conferred Honorary Doctorate *"Doctor of Science"* by the Rajiv Gandhi University of Health Sciences (RGUHS) for his contribution to society in the field of ophthalmology during the 16th Annual Convocation of RGUHS in March 2014.

He has also received many awards at various academic conferences and has publications in national and international peer-reviewed journals.

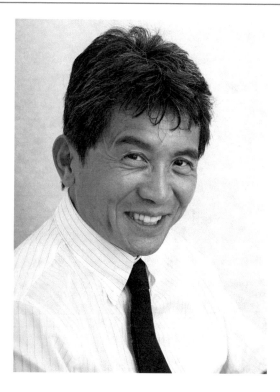

Kimiya Shimizu received an M.D. in ophthalmology from Kitasato University School of Medicine in 1976 and a Ph.D. in ophthalmology from Tokyo University in 1984. From 1985 to 1998, he worked as a director of Musashino Red Cross Hospital. He is currently a professor and chairman of ophthalmology at Kitasato University School of Medicine, where he specializes in cataract and refractive surgery.

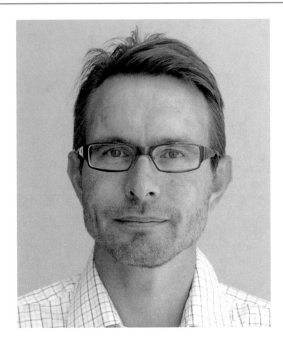

Anders Ivarsen is consultant and assistant professor within the cornea and refractive section in the Department of Ophthalmology in Aarhus, Denmark.

He received his Ph.D. on refractive surgery in 2004. He has been working actively in the field of refractive surgery since 2000 and started performing SMILE procedures as early as 2011.

Anders Ivarsen has participated in several studies on SMILE and has contributed to more than 10 papers on refractive lenticule extraction.

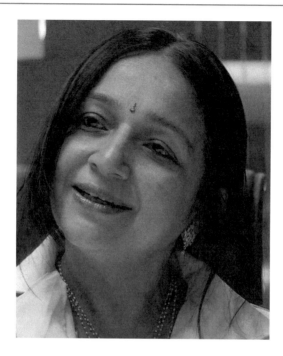

Rupal Shah is the Group Medical Director, New Vision Laser Centers-Centre for Sight, a leading chain of vision correction centers in India. She has been a pioneer of various vision correction techniques. She was the first person to perform single-incision ReLEx and SMILE procedures in the world. Over 1200 ophthalmologists have performed their first LASIK, Femto-LASIK, or SMILE procedures under her mentorship. She has performed surgery at more than 30 different locations around the world. She practices in both Vadodara and Mumbai, India. She has several publications in peer-reviewed journals and has written many book chapters.

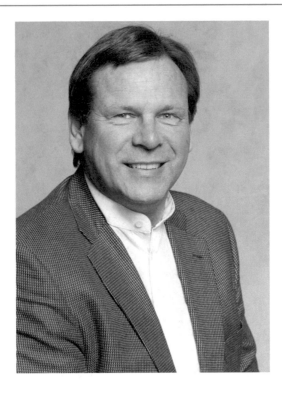

Bertram Meyer is a specialist in laser refractive surgery since 1992 and has performed SMILE procedures since 2010. He works in private clinics in Cologne and in Dubai. He has given continuous and regular lectures and updates during the annual meetings of DOG, DOC, DGII, and European Society of Cataract and Refractive Surgeons (ESCRS) about Femto-Lasik and ReLEx® SMILE. He has been a member of the Advisory Board for Refractive Laser Surgery for Carl Zeiss Meditec for many years.

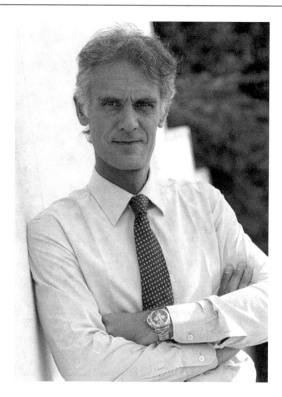

Jose L. Güell is Founding Partner of IMO and Director of the Cornea and Refractive Surgery Department. He is Associate Professor of Ophthalmology at the Autonoma University of Barcelona, Scientific Coordinator and Professor of the Anterior Segment activities at the European School for Advanced Studies in Ophthalmology (ESASO), Lugano, Past President of EuCornea (European Society of Cornea and Surface Disease), and Specialist and Past President of the ESCRS. He has published around 190 articles on corneal surgery and diseases and refractive surgery in national and international journals and has given lectures around the world during the last 20 years.

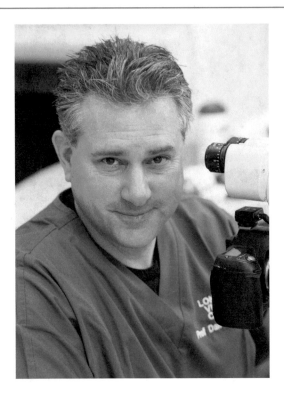

Dan Z. Reinstein is the Medical Director of London Vision Clinic, Adjunct Professor of Ophthalmology at Columbia University Medical Center, New York, and Professeur Associe en Ophtalmologie at the Centre Hospitalier National d'Ophtalmologie des Quinze-Vingts, Paris. He is a graduate of Cambridge University. Professor Reinstein's research focuses on using Artemis VHF digital ultrasound to improve refractive surgery, in particular using the corneal epithelium for keratoconus screening and therapeutic corneal refractive surgery. He is also the lead consultant to Carl Zeiss Meditec, for whom he has developed Laser Blended Vision for correcting presbyopia and has contributed to the development of ReLEx® SMILE. His research has led to over 115 peer-reviewed publications, 30 book chapters, and 500 international presentations and lectures. He was awarded the Waring Medal in 2006 and received the Kritzinger Award in 2013.

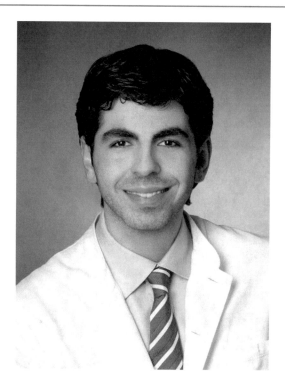

Apostolos Lazaridis is a specialist of Ophthalmology at the first Department of Ophthalmology of the National and Kapodistrian University of Athens, Greece and a research associate at the Department of Ophthalmology, Philipps University of Marburg, Germany. Dr. Lazaridis studied Medicine in Aristotle University of Thessaloniki, Greece. After a clinical traineeship in Ophthalmology at the University of Berlin (Charité Campus Virchow), he started his ophthalmology residency training at Ophthalmology Clinic Dr. Georg, Bad Rothenfelde, Germany and continued as research fellow at the Institute of Experimental Ophthalmology, University of Münster, Germany. Dr. Lazaridis completed his residency training and dissertation at the Department of Ophthalmology, Philipps University of Marburg, Germany. He became a board-certified ophthalmologist in 2014 and a fellow of the European Board of Ophthalmology (FEBO) in 2015. His clinical, surgical and research activity focuses on corneal refractive surgery, keratoplasty, keratoconus and corneal wound healing.

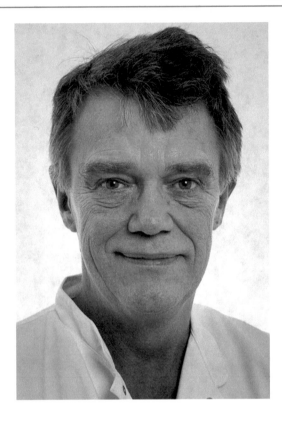

Jesper Hjortdal is Clinical Professor and Consultant at the Department of Ophthalmology, Aarhus University Hospital. He graduated from Aarhus University in 1988 and started basic and clinical research in corneal optics, biomechanics, and refractive surgery in 1990. In 1992 he was Visiting Research Associate at Stanford University, USA. He completed his PhD study in 1995 and became Doctor of Medicine in 1998. In 1998, Jesper Hjortdal finished specialists training in Ophthalmology and was in 2000-2001 Honorary Fellow to the Cornea and External Diseases at Moorfields Eye Hospital, London. Jesper Hjortdal is president for the Danish Ophthalmological Society for the European Eye Bank Association.

Jesper Hjortdal has published more than 130 papers. In 2013 he received the Waring Medal for Editorial Excellence (best paper in Journal of Refractive Surgery 2012).

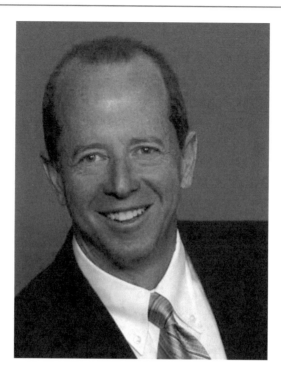

Jon Dishler, MD, FACS, is an American Board Certified Ophthalmologist who is recognized for his contributions to refractive surgery for over 30 years. Awarded numerous patents and publications, Dr. Dishler also built one of the first FDA approved excimer laser systems. He has been a clinical investigator for multiple FDA trials, most recently as the US Medical Monitor for the SMILE procedure. Jon has contributed both as a clinical site and scientific consultant on this project. Dr. Dishler realized that the lenticules removed in the SMILE procedure provided a unique opportunity to study the femtosecond laser tissue interaction in humans. With the help of co-authors, sample tissue was imaged using a new method of scanning electron microscopy (eSEM), the results of which are presented in this text.

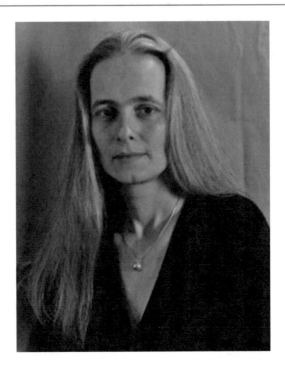

Kathleen S. Kunert is senior consultant at the Eye Hospital, Helios Klinikum Erfurt, and holds a position as professor of clinical optometry at the University of Applied Sciences Ernst-Abbe Jena in cooperation with ZVA Knechtsteden. She obtained her degree in human medicine from the Universität Leipzig in 1996 followed by a 3 year postdoctoral fellowship at the Schepens Eye Research Institute and Cornea Department of Ophthalmology, Harvard Medical School, Boston, USA. In 2005, she qualified as a specialist for ophthalmology and was trained at the University Eye Hospital Charité, Campus Virchow, Berlin, and the Eye Hospital, Helios Klinikum Erfurt.

She published numerous papers with special focus on dry eye, ocular allergy, femtosecond laser systems used for refractive correction of different eye diseases, and studies on accommodation and presbyopia.

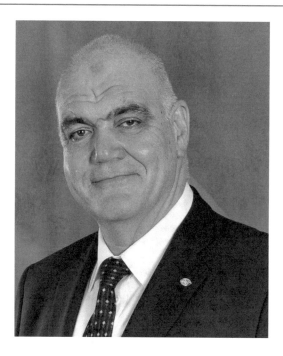

Ibrahim Osama is a clinical Professor of Ophthalmology and Immediate Past President of Alexandria University, being the first elected president (2011–2014). He completed a Fellowship in Corneal and Refractive Surgery at Emory Eye Clinic, USA, and was chief of Corneal and Refractive Unit, Magrabi Eye Centers, Saudi Arabia. He supervised and discussed more than 70 master's and doctoral theses for 30 years and promoted refractive surgery all over the Arab world and the Middle East, helping establish many centers. He is an active member of almost all prestigious ophthalmic societies in the world. He has been actively involved as a principal investigator and consultant for many clinical studies and research projects. He is the recipient of MEACO Distinction Award for 2012, Lifetime Achievement Award by the American Academy of Ophthalmology (AAO, 2013), and Casebeer Award by the International Society of Refractive Surgery (ISRS, 2012).

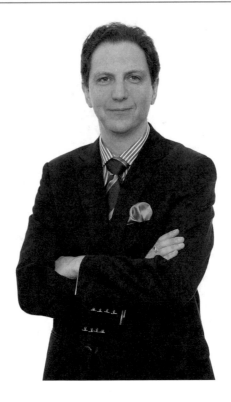

Walter Sekundo is Professor and Chairman, Department of Ophthalmology, Philipps University of Marburg, Germany. He studied Medicine in Frankfurt (Germany), New Orleans, and Durham (USA). He was a resident at the University of Bonn in Germany and a Fellow in Corneal and Refractive Surgery at Moorfields Eye Hospital (UK) and Ocular Pathology at the University of Glasgow, UK. He also holds a degree of "Health Care Manager." Prof. Sekundo has published over 100 original papers, over 25 book chapters, and given over 300 presentations at national and international meetings. He is a reviewer for 11 ophthalmic journals and a Board Member of "Der Ophthalmologe." Prof. Sekundo has performed over 20,000 surgical procedures in the entire field of ophthalmology and has been repeatedly named as one of the 30 top eye surgeons in Germany. He was the first surgeon in the world to have performed FLEx and SMILE.

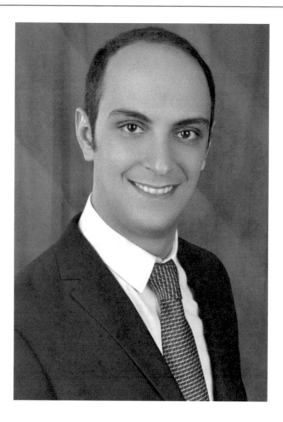

Moones Fathi Abdalla works as medical and research director of the International Femto-Lasik Centre (IFLC), Dusit Thani Lakeveiw, Cairo. He is also employed as refractive surgery consultant and surgeon trainer at Royal Vision Center, Alexandria, and cornea and refractive consultant at Cornea Center, Alexandria. Moones Fathi Abdalla started performing SMILE since 2010. He has performed over 7000 SMILE procedures, trained more than 35 surgeons in doing SMILE, and contributed in many studies concerning SMILE.

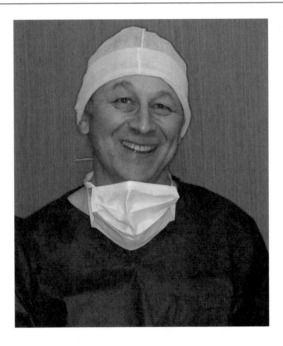

Jean-François Faure is an ophthalmologist specialized in laser refractive surgery (myopia, hyperopia, astigmatism, and presbyopia), cataract surgery, glaucoma surgery, eyelid surgery, and botulinum toxin injections in the treatment of blepharospasm and wrinkle correction.

He is a member of the following Scientific Societies:

SFO (French Society of Ophthalmology)

ASCRS (American Society of Cataract and Refractive Surgery)

ESCRS (European Society of Cataract and Refractive Surgery)

SAFIR (French Society of Intraocular Implants and Refractive Surgery)

EUCORNEA (European Society of Cornea and Ocular Surface Disease Specialists)

Part I

Basic Principles

Femtosecond Laser Keratomes for Small Incision Lenticule Extraction (SMILE)

Mark Bischoff and Gregor Strobrawa

Contents

Back in 2002 when we began developing the technology for vision correction by means of lenticule extraction at ZEISS, many experts still considered such a corrective procedure impossible. Their skepticism was not unfounded.

If one considers that in ablative procedures (LASIK, PRK) a layer of tissue approximately 1 µm thick is ablated with a single pulse from a medical excimer laser, it is difficult to imagine, at first, how a lenticule could be prepared inside the cornea with comparable precision using a femtosecond laser keratome. After all, the axial length of the femtosecond laser focus (Rayleigh length) is several micrometers and is therefore too long for the desired machining accuracy, at first glance. Fortunately, this assessment is based on a flawed logic, which we aim to illustrate in this chapter. We shall also present important features of lenticule extraction in comparison with LASIK and PRK. Where we feel it important for the clinicians' understanding of the basic physico-technical principles, we shall also go into more detail on the technical features of laser therapy equipment.

M. Bischoff (✉) • G. Strobrawa
R&D Refractive Lasers, Carl Zeiss Meditec AG, Jena, Germany
e-mail: mark.bischoff@zeiss.com; gregor.strobrawa@zeiss.com

© Springer International Publishing Switzerland 2015
W. Sekundo (ed.), *Small Incision Lenticule Extraction (SMILE):
Principles, Techniques, Complication Management, and Future Concepts*,
DOI 10.1007/978-3-319-18530-9_1

The application of laser light has a long tradition in ophthalmology. The first treatments for posterior capsular opacification, also known as "secondary cataract" (laser posterior capsulotomy), were performed back in 1979 using a pulsed infrared laser. In these procedures, which are still commonly used today, a short infrared laser pulse is focused on the target area behind the intraocular lens, where a resulting local plasma bubble within the eye tissue causes the disruption of the posterior capsular bag. The pulse length is typically several nanoseconds (approx. 4 ns) and is therefore around 10,000 times longer than the pulse from a femtosecond laser keratome. In the 1980s, the technology for creating ultrashort light pulses underwent dramatic development. The femtosecond lasers available as a result enabled not only a vast number of very significant scientific findings, but also a range of new medical laser applications. However, it was not until the development of compact and cost-efficient ultrashort pulse lasers based on diode-pumped solid-state lasers that such lasers became suitable for use in everyday medical devices. By as early as the end of the 1980s, the idea emerged to combine the local effect of focused infrared laser pulses inside the eye with the automatic laser beam control, for which scanning excimer lasers were known. In 2001, IntraLase, Inc. (Irvine, USA) launched the first femtosecond laser keratome. This enabled computer-assisted, automated scanning of individual plasma bubbles into lines and surfaces, thus allowing precise incisions to be created inside the cornea.

A flap incision requires the laminar alignment of about one million plasma bubbles. Each of the ultrashort laser pulses first creates a plasma at the site of its focus, thus breaking down the tissue material there (primary effect). The plasma then expands, resulting in a gas bubble, which stretches and mechanically separates surrounding tissue structures [1]. This separation often proceeds along lamellar structures of the tissue, similar to tissue cleaving. This secondary effect of tissue cleaving is all the more pronounced the higher the pulse energy. When responding to the question posed at the beginning of this chapter, as to the precision with which tissue separation occurs, the underlying mechanism must be considered. According to this mechanism, it is not a single laser pulse that creates an incision in the tissue, but, rather, the collective effect of 10,000–100,000 pulses per square millimeter. It is therefore clear that the Rayleigh length as a characteristic measurement of the axial length of a single laser focus cannot be interpreted as the axial cutting precision of a femtosecond laser keratome. The axial cutting precision results – contrary to what was presumed at first glance – from the averaging of the axial precision of a very large number of individual laser pulses. Ultimately, the very good clinical results leave no doubt about the adequacy of cutting precision.

From a physico-technical perspective, one is inclined to further distinguish the feature of a tissue incision inadequately termed "precision." Possible characteristics include "contour accuracy" and "roughness." These two parameters are also more suitable for comparisons with the ablation behavior of excimer lasers or femtosecond laser keratomes with each other (Fig. 1.1).

The ablation behavior of excimer lasers is characterized, for example, by a particularly low surface roughness. Even state-of-the-art femtosecond laser keratomes now achieve a low roughness with low pulse energy and higher spot density (number of

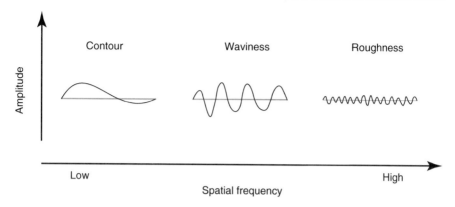

Fig. 1.1 Contour deviation and roughness are useful parameters for characterizing a cut surface. They measure deviations of the intended shape with very low and very high spatial frequency. Deviations with intermediate spatial frequency may be interpreted as "waviness"

spots per surface area). For a lenticule with a diameter of 7 mm, for example, each of the cut surfaces is prepared at a spot distance of 3 μm by almost 4.3 million laser shots. One should compare this with around 100 shots from an excimer laser, which produce the same surface covering. If one imagines the "filling" of a surface with these shot patterns with very different densities, intuitively one knows that any deviations when working with an excimer laser will show up as waviness. Height errors in the created profile therefore change only slowly with the position (technical term: low spatial frequencies). The characteristic "contour deviation" is used to describe a limit case of the lowest spatial frequencies. A lack of contour accuracy causes in particular an error in the correction of sphere, cylinder, and spherical aberration. The granularity of the scan pattern causes in particular roughness and waviness. With excimer laser ablation, however, there are further possible sources of error. These include the characteristics of the ambient air and the tissue to be ablated. The iterative character of the ablation process of an excimer laser leads to the summation of these errors during the procedure, which, when compounded, therefore increases with the magnitude of the planned refractive correction. The influence of these sources of error accordingly grows with the depth of ablation and the size of the optical zone.

In the SMILE procedure, however, the magnitude of correction has no direct influence on absolute precision. Ultimately, therefore, it makes almost no difference whether the correction magnitude is 1 D or 10 D. At second glance, however, it becomes evident that this procedure can result, in the case of very minor corrections (<1 D), in an interaction between the two incisions, which are very close to each other in a minor correction (cap incision and lenticule incision, Fig. 1.3). If this is to be avoided, minimizing the gas bubbles and thus using as low a pulse energy as possible is beneficial in terms of the quality of the procedure. The comparison of the femtosecond laser keratomes available on the market concerning pulse energy thus also gives an initial indication of their fundamental suitability for lenticule preparation. A first attempt by IntraLase to perform a refractive correction by preparing a stromal tissue disk was reported, however, seemed not pursued any further by consecutive clinical trials [2].

1.1 Why Does the Pulse Energy Used by the Femtosecond Laser Keratomes Vary?

It is not possible to set the pulse energy for a particular femtosecond laser keratome as low as desired. The minimum pulse energy of each of these systems is determined by its ability to generate the necessary radiation intensity for plasma formation in the beam focus (pulse energy per focus area). One can also imagine this intensity as the photon density in the medium, which must be reached so that the tissue that is transparent under normal condition absorbs enough radiation (nonlinear) for all chemical bonds to be broken and plasma to form in the laser focus. The idea is therefore to concentrate as many photons as possible in as small a volume of space as possible at the same time. This is achieved by extreme focusing of

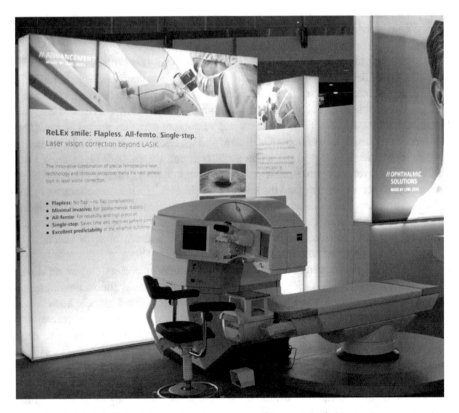

Fig. 1.2 The VisuMax® femtosecond laser keratome. It utilizes full-field objective lenses to provide maximum cutting precision, efficiency, and comfort (Source: ZEISS, 2012 at WOC Abu Dhabi)

ultrashort pulses. The focus volume decreases as the beam cone angle increases, the largest possible beam cone angle favors the achievement of plasma formation at the lowest possible pulse energy. In optical engineering, it is common to use the term "numerical aperture" instead of beam cone angle (angle of aperture) (Fig. 1.2).

Today's femtosecond laser keratomes can be divided into two categories, which are distinguished by the optical systems they use. The first is the class of devices with full-field objective lenses, which include, e.g., IntraLase and VisuMax. The second category includes the devices made by Ziemer, which work with partial-field objective lenses and which can only address a small section of the actual treatment field, without moving the objective. Whereas in the case of the really large full-field objective lenses a high numerical aperture (large beam cone angle) is quite costly, and, in addition, the human anatomy presents certain limitations (nose, cheekbone), a partial-field objective lens is comparatively small and cost-effective. One "gains" this cost advantage with the partial-field objective lens, but with less freedom when it comes to shaping the cutting surfaces. Partial-field objective lens systems therefore tend to be unsuitable for lenticule preparation. In addition to a suitable objective lens, an appropriate beam control is also required in order to also be able to achieve the dome-shaped incision curvature necessary for lenticule preparation with the required precision.

1.2   What Shapes Are the Incisions for a SMILE Lenticule and What Precision Is Required?

The shape of the incisions in lenticule preparation is based equally on the basic principles of the initial pioneering work of José I. Barraquer Moner in 1948 [3], the theoretical work of Munnerlyn et al. in 1988 [4], and early work of Swinger et al. and Lai [5, 6] on intrastromal cutting. It is also based on the work of ZEISS on the specific technical execution, which we have been developing in collaboration with our colleagues since 2002 [7–9]. The experiences with LASIK and PRK played a rather subordinate role in this, because the transferability of empirical knowledge concerning the specific shape of the ablation profiles in these two procedures is not really given for various reasons. Furthermore, there is the clinical methodology, which began with the pioneering work of Sekundo and Blum [10] and was then gradually improved. A great many outstanding refractive surgeons contributed to this, some of whom also appear in this book with their own contribution.

Let us turn now to the current conventional design of the incision technique for lenticule preparation. Figure 1.3 shows the main features of the now conventional incisions created in the SMILE procedure. The cap cut is always made parallel to the corneal surface and can vary in thickness (for more information, see Chap. 12). The refractive effect results from the interplay between the cap cut and the deeper lenticule cut. The latter is performed first by the laser keratome to avoid a shadowing effect of the laser beam due to bubbles in incisions above. Both incisions are connected to each other by a side cut on the edge of the lenticule, which is normally

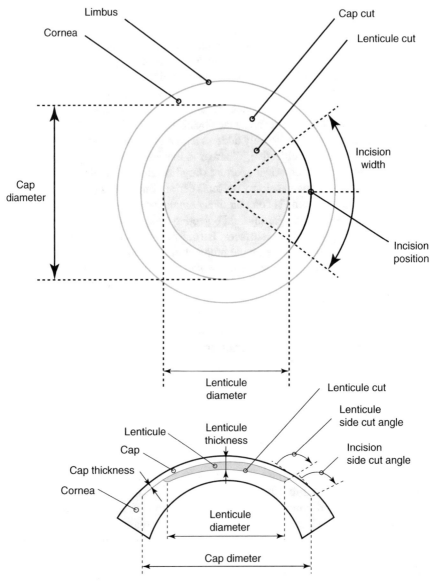

Fig. 1.3 Parameters associated with SMILE for myopia. (**a**) Is a schematic view from above of a cornea with lenticule and cap already cut. (**b**) Is side view the same. Many parameters can be selected directly by the user, such as the opening incision width, the lenticule diameter, the cap thickness, the minimum lenticule thickness, the cap diameter, and the cap and lenticule side cut angles. Other parameters, such as the lenticule thickness and residual bed thickness and shape of the lenticule (not labeled), are calculated by the VisuMax Laser Keratome software based upon the manifest and target refraction values and preoperative corneal curvature entered by the user (Note that the aspect ratio has been modified in this illustration.)

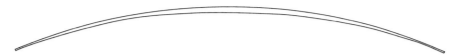

Fig. 1.4 A cross section of a typical lenticule for a correction of myopia, shown with the correct aspect ratio, but with the scale approximately 25:1 for clarity (sphere=−5 diopters, cylinder=0 diopters, diameter=6 mm, minimum lenticule thickness=15 μm, side cut angle=90°). Note that the curvatures are as shown and that the lenticule is not cut with either flat or with parallel surfaces

approx. 10–15 μm in length. The side cut has been clinically proven, because it increases the surgeon's control over the completeness of the lenticule extraction. The parallel position of the cap cut with the front of the cornea also proves to be very advantageous in the rare cases of complications (suction loss) or follow-up corrections, as well as in respect of the biomechanical stability of the cornea. Today, the majority of surgeons practicing the SMILE procedure do so with just a single access incision (2–4 mm) to the front of the cornea (also see Chaps. 5 and 10).

In order to clearly present various important characteristics, drawings of lenticules are almost always elongated in the axial direction (optical axis) (e.g., Fig. 1.3). One should not get a false impression of the reality, however. Figure 1.4 illustrates with a real aspect ratio the very subtle structure of a typical lenticule.

In addition to the spherical correction, the vision correction also often involves correction of astigmatism (for clinical results, see Chap. 8). For the lenticule cut, this means that the incision must be ellipsoidal in shape, rather than spherical. In such cases, the surgeon can observe, when making the incision, elliptical spiral pathways being scanned in the lenticule incision, rather than the usual circular spiral pathways. These are the contour lines of the respective ellipsoid. The initial elliptical elongation of the lenticule that results is transformed back to a circular edge by means of a special transition zone, which is completed with the side cut. The dependence of the lenticule thickness on the amount of refractive correction follows the above-mentioned theoretical limit value according to Munnerlyn, whereby the rule of thumb is: 1 D correction at the 6 mm zone corresponds to around 13 μm tissue thickness. In myopia correction, this measurement presents as the central thickness of the lenticule; in hyperopia correction, it presents as the thickness of the lenticule at the edge of the optical zone. The total thickness of the lenticule is calculated by adding the minimum thickness of the lenticule of 10–15 μm, which, in a quick comparison with an excimer laser, suggests a slightly higher tissue removal of the SMILE procedure compared with LASIK or PRK. However, it must be considered that the tissue ablation, in addition to the linear dependency on the correction value, shows a quadratic dependency on the diameter of the optical zone. This gives rise to the question concerning the parameter to be used for a suitable comparison between SMILE and LASIK, for the lateral extension of the optical zone. One might come to different conclusions in this respect. Ultimately, however, the only matter of interest in everyday clinical practice is whether a patient obtains the best possible

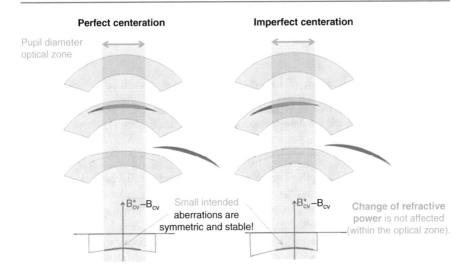

Fig. 1.5 The optical effect of a rotational decentration of the lenticule inside the stroma is similar to a shifting contact lens. This is due to the general method as well as the design of the cut surfaces in the ReLEx® software. In the figure the induced change of refractive power (B^*_{CV}–B_{CV}) is shown not to be sensitive for decentration of a SMILE treatment. The optical zone (*green*) and the corneal volume (*gray*) are shown in the preoperative state (*top*), with lenticule cut (*middle*) and with lenticule extracted (*bottom*). Perfect centration is shown on the left-hand side, and an example of decentration is shown on the right-hand side

refractive correction right across the entire optical zone delivering good vision under all relevant light conditions, without unnecessarily impairing the stability of the cornea. In this respect, there is no doubt that SMILE offers certain advantages over the conventional procedures (Fig. 1.5) [11].

1.3 Centering Accuracy

We are often asked whether the centering accuracy typically achieved by the clinicians on the VisuMax device is sufficient in the SMILE procedure. While the clinical data on centration after SMILE are presented in Chap. 14, let us explain the theoretical background. Indeed, this question is quite justified, because the clinical experience of many clinicians with LASIK and PRK is that there is a risk, in both LASIK and PRK, of clinically relevant higher-order aberrations being induced due to decentration. There is an essential difference with lenticule preparation for SMILE. The decentration of a lenticule induces a comparatively small amount of higher-order aberrations. The reason for this quite different behavior of lenticule extraction and ablation procedures (LASIK, PRK) lies in the above-described sensitivity of excimer ablation compared with the variable characteristics of the tissue. In other words, where there is decentration of the excimer laser ablation, higher-order aberrations will always be induced. This is mainly due to ablation errors around the edge of the working area, which arise due to distortion (projection errors) and variation of the ablation efficiency. These effects, which can only be partly controlled in LASIK and PRK, even with state-of-the-art excimer lasers, are entirely excluded with the SMILE procedure. Besides a comparatively more favorable biomechanical situation, this definitely contributes to the very good predictability of refractive correction in the SMILE procedure.

In this chapter, we have touched upon a number of physico-technical issues and have explained, insofar as possible within this scope, how and why the SMILE procedure works technically. We have also explained why a lenticule can be created with sufficient cutting precision, what shape it is, and with what level of centering accuracy it must be prepared within the tissue. The next chapter looks at the fascinating biomedical processes in the patient's cornea, which are triggered by the creation and extraction of a lenticule.

References

1. Riau AK, Poh R, Pickard DS, Park CHJ, Chaurasia SS, Metha JS (2014) Nanoscale helium ion microscopic analysis of collagen fiber changes following femtosecond laser dissection of human cornea. J Biomed Nanotechnol 10:1552–1562
2. Ratkay-Traub I, Ferincz IE, Juhasz T, Kurtz RM, Krueger RR (2003) First clinical results with the femtosecond neodymium-glass laser in refractive surgery. J Refract Surg 19:94–103
3. Barraquer J (1949) Queratoplastia refractiva. Estud Inform Oftalmol 10:2–21
4. Munnerlyn CR, Koons SI, Marshall J (1988) Photorefractive keratectomy: a technique for laser refractive surgery. J Cataract Refract Surg 14(1):46–52
5. Swinger CA, Krumeich JH, Cassiday D (1986) Planar lamellar refractive keratoplasty. J Refract Surg 2(1):17–24
6. Lai ST. Ophthalmic surgical laser and method. US 5,984,916 (filed 1993)
7. Bendett M, Bischoff M, Gerlach M, Muehlhoff D Apparatus and method for ophthalmologic surgical procedures using a femtosecond fiber laser. US 7,131,968 (filed 2003)
8. Muehlhoff D, Gerlach M, Sticker M, Lang C, Bischoff M, Bergt M Device for forming curved cuts in a transparent material. EP 1648360 (filed 2004)
9. Bischoff M, Sticker M, Stobrawa G Behandlungsvorrichtung zur operative Fehlsichtigkeitskorrektur eines Auges. DE102006053120 (filed 2006)
10. Sekundo W, Kunert K, Russmann C, Gille A, Bissmann W, Stobrawa G, Sticker M, Bischoff M, Blum M (2008) First efficacy and safety study of femtosecond lenticule extraction for the correction of myopia: six-month results. J Cataract Refract Surg 34(9):1513–1520
11. Reinstein DZ, Archer TJ, Randleman J (2013) Bradley's mathematical model to compare the relative tensile strength of the cornea after PRK, LASIK, and small incision lenticule extraction. J Cataract Refract Surg 29(7):454–460

Wound Healing After ReLEx® Surgery

Yu-Chi Liu, Donald T-H Tan, and Jodhbir S. Mehta

Contents

2.1 Basic Principles of Femtosecond Laser

The femtosecond laser consists of a solid-state laser source that emits impulses of wavelength close to the infrared spectrum and of duration measurable in femtoseconds [1]. The definition of a femtosecond is 10^{-15} s. Unlike photoablation generated by a 193 um wavelength of light from an argon fluoride excimer laser, the 1,053 um wavelength of light used by the femtosecond laser produces a

Y.-C. Liu • D.T.-H. Tan • J.S. Mehta (✉)
Tissue Engineering and Stem Cells Group, Singapore Eye Research Institute,
Singapore, Singapore

Corneal and External Eye Disease Service, Singapore National Eye Centre,
Singapore, Singapore

Department of Clinical Sciences, Duke-NUS Graduate Medical School,
Singapore, Singapore
e-mail: liuchiy@gmail.com; donald.tan.t.h@snec.com.sg; jodmehta@yahoo.com

© Springer International Publishing Switzerland 2015
W. Sekundo (ed.), *Small Incision Lenticule Extraction (SMILE):*
Principles, Techniques, Complication Management, and Future Concepts,
DOI 10.1007/978-3-319-18530-9_2

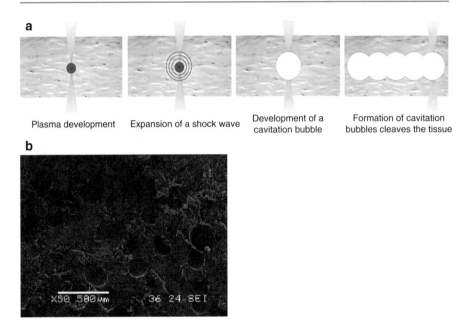

Fig. 2.1 (a) Illustration of photodisruption process in corneal stroma. (b) Scanning electron microscopic micrograph showing the cavitation bubbles generated during the photodisruption process

different tissue interaction, known as photodisruption. During the photodisruption process, plasma (free electrons and ions), an acoustic shockwave, thermal energy, and then a cavitation bubble are created [2] (Fig. 2.1). This process of photodisruption, termed laser-induced optical breakdown, essentially vaporizes a small volume of tissue [3]. The threshold for photodisruption is inversely related to the laser's intensity. The shorter the pulse's duration, the smaller the diameter of the laser spot, the lower the energy needed for photodisruption. The femtosecond laser permits the creation of corneal cuts of different shapes, at desired depths, but the fundamental requirement for this is corneal transparency that allows precise focus of the laser spots [1]. The corneal surface is the reference plane for the laser. A lens with a higher numerical aperture will create a more focal laser spot in terms of its diameter and volume, which enhances the depth accuracy and overall precision of the lamellar cut. The VisuMax® system (Carl Zeiss Meditec AG, Jena, Germany) used for refractive lenticule extraction (ReLEx®), uses a high numerical aperture lens [4], with lower pulse energy and higher pulse frequency (500 kHz) [5]. Lower pulse energy is generally associated with fewer unwanted side effects, such as an opaque bubble layer, collateral thermal damage, corneal inflammation, and diffuse lamellar keratitis as well as transient light sensitivity [6–8].

2.2   Wound Healing After Refractive Lenticule Extraction (ReLEx®)

Corneal wound healing has an important effect on the safety, efficacy, and stability of laser vision correction [9, 10]. Biological differences in wound-healing responses are thought to be a major factor affecting the predictability of refractive surgery in some patients (overcorrection, undercorrection, regression, and irregular astigmatism) [9]. Corneal wound healing has also been reported to be associated with corneal haze, myopia regression, and epithelial ingrowth after femtosecond laser in situ keratomileusis (Fs-LASIK) [11–13].

Corneal wound healing involves a complex cascade of pathways. On the molecular and cellular level, cytokines and growth factors, such as interleukin (IL)-1, tumor necrosis factor (TNF)-α, epidermal growth factor, and platelet-derived growth factor, are released from the injured epithelium [14–16]. This injury can take the form of an incision, femtosecond laser exposure, or other insults [10]. The released cytokines and growth factors mediate stromal keratocytes apoptosis [17], followed by proliferation and migration of remaining stromal keratocytes within a few hours to restore stromal cellularity [18, 19]. Within 24 h, inflammatory cells migrate to phagocytize the apoptotic cells and enhance the transformation of keratocytes to fibroblasts [10]. Transforming growth factor-β (TGF-β) and other cytokines then induce the differentiation of fibroblasts to myofibroblasts [19], and the appearance of myofibroblasts is the primary biological event associated with the development of corneal surface irregularity and corneal haze [20, 21] (Fig. 2.2). During the corneal wound-healing response, the balance between myofibroblast precursor apoptosis and myofibroblast development is a critical determinate of whether corneal haze develops [22]. Moreover, corneal avascularity, or the maintenance of a corneal "angiogenic privilege" state, is important for corneal transparency [23, 24]. The maintenance of corneal avascularity depends on a fine balance between the production of angiogenic and anti-angiogeneic factors [9]. One of the first molecules thought to have a major role in maintaining corneal avascularity was pigment epithelium-derived factor (PEDF) [25].

2.2.1   Corneal Wound Healing and Inflammatory Response After ReLEx®: Animal Study

There are only a few studies investigating the corneal wound healing and inflammatory response after ReLEx in the literature. Our group has investigated and compared the early corneal wound repair and inflammatory responses after FLEx and Fs-LASIK 1 day after surgery [26]. We demonstrated that (1) the expression of fibronectin, which is produced by activated keratocytes and plays an important role in cell adhesion, growth, migration, and differentiation during the corneal wound-healing process [27], showed a less abundant expression around the incision line in the corneas

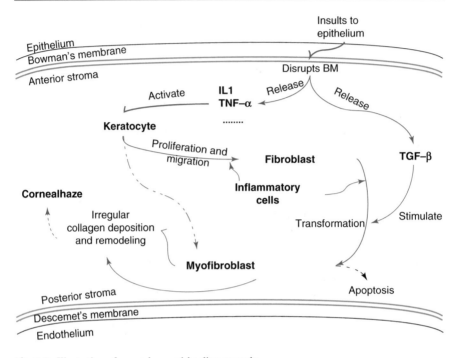

Fig. 2.2 Illustration of corneal wound-healing cascade

that underwent FLEx than Fs-LASIK. The differences became more marked as the power of correction was increased. This was because the higher energy of the excimer laser in Fs-LASIK caused an elevated intensity of fibronectin staining. Also in Fs-LASIK, a wider treatment zone including a 1.0-mm blend zone is performed (a conventional blend zone is not needed in ReLEx®). A similar trend was also seen in the number of CD11b-positive cells (a marker of monocytes) that play a role in inflammatory infiltration after injury. The results suggested that excimer laser treatment in Fs-LASIK stimulated a higher degree of inflammation. Furthermore, we found that there were no CD11b-positive cells seen along the laser vertical or lamellar cutting plane in the post-FLEx corneas when the lenticule was not removed. This indicated that the inflammatory response following ReLEx mainly comes from the surgical dissection, rather than the laser. (2) TUNEL-positive cells (indicating apoptotic cells) were detected in the corneal center and periphery of flap, suggesting femtosecond laser energy still induced keratocyte cell death in the absence of injured epithelium. There was no significant disparity in the number of apoptotic cells between Fs-LASIK group and ReLEx, although more apoptotic cells were observed in Fs-LASIK group. (3) Ki-67, a cell proliferation marker, was primarily present in the epithelial cells of the flap margin, rather than the epithelium of cornea center, for both groups. This indicated the proliferation activity was mainly seen in the areas where epithelium was damaged or displaced. No significant difference in the Ki-67 expression around the flap margin was observed between two groups.

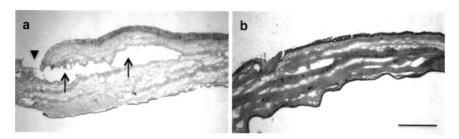

Fig. 2.3 Light microscopic cross-sectional histologic specimen in rabbit corneas stained by hematoxylin-eosin (H & E) stain showing the small incision (*arrowhead*) and lamellar dissection wound (*arrows*) were observed at day 1 postoperatively (**a**) but almost healed at week 1 postoperatively (**b**). Original magnification: 100×, scale bar 100 μm

Dong et al. [28] evaluated and compared the early corneal wound healing and inflammatory response after SMILE versus Fs-LASIK using a rabbit model. The authors reported that (1) TUNEL-positive cells were detected at the lamellar interface after SMILE and Fs-LASIK procedures at postoperative 4 and 24 h. A statistically significantly fewer TUNEL-positive stromal cells were observed in the SMILE group than in the Fs-LASIK group at postoperative 4 and 24 h. (2) There were statistically significantly fewer Ki67-positive cells in the stroma in the SMILE group as compared to the Fs-LASIK group, at day 3 and week 1 postoperatively, indicating that SMILE stimulated less stromal keratocyte proliferation. (3) The CD11b-positive cells were significantly less in the SMILE group at day 1, day 3, and week 1 postoperatively. The authors postulated this could be due to the following reasons: a small incision for SMILE produced fewer cytokines to attract inflammatory cells in the injury, the intrastromal dissection by a femtosecond laser contributed to less extent of tissue injury compared with the stromal ablation by an excimer laser, and there was less necrotic debris in the interface after SMILE.

Our group has also studied the early corneal wound-healing inflammatory response following SMILE in a rabbit model. The small vertical incision and lamellar dissection wounds were observed at day 1 (Fig. 2.3a), but both of them almost healed at week 1 postoperatively (Fig. 2.3b). The CD11b-positive cells were apparent at 1 day postoperatively, more abundant around the vertical incision site (Fig. 2.4a) than the lamellar incision plane (Fig. 2.4b). This is understandable since the vertical incision cuts through the epithelium and basement membrane. In healthy and intact corneas, the basement membrane can function to bind cytokines [29], suggesting that it may act as a physical barrier for signaling molecules that are produced by the epithelial cells or tear fluid [30]. Thus, when the barrier is compromised, the underlying stroma is exposed to the signaling molecules, and the inflammatory cell infiltration is augmented. Moreover, the surgical manipulations around the incision, such as inserting instruments via the small incision to dissect the anterior and posterior surfaces of the lenticule and to extract the lenticule, might elicit cytokines to attract inflammatory cells because of more disturbances on the basement membrane. It might be also due to the some inadvertent minor epithelial abrasions or small tears at the incision

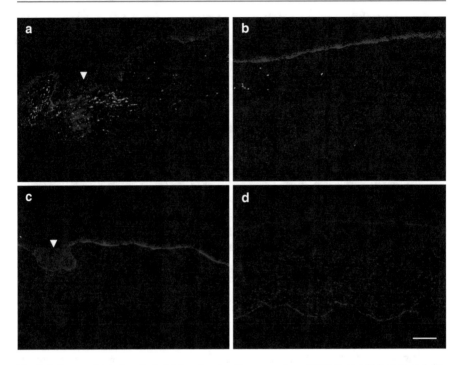

Fig. 2.4 Immunohistochemical staining showing the expression of CD11b in rabbit corneas 1 day (**a, b**) and 1 week (**c, d**) at the incision (**a, c**; *arrowheads*) and extracted lenticule plane (**b, d**) after −4.0 D SMILE. The CD11b-positive cells were apparent at 1 day, more abundant around the incision (**a**) than around the lamellar cutting plane (**b**) and significantly reduced at 1 week postoperatively (**c, d**). Original magnification: 200×, scale bar 100 μm

site, which have been reported to be a common postoperative complication after SMILE [31]. At 1 week postoperatively, the CD11b expression was significantly reduced (Figs. 2.4c and 2.4d). This observation was different from what was reported by Dong et al. [28]. They showed an increase in CD11b-positive cells in the central cornea at 1 week compared to 1 day postoperatively. However, CD11b is an early inflammatory marker expressed on the surface of neutrophils, monoctyes, and macrophages, which have been reported to be attracted to the wound site within 24 h and be replaced by lymphocytes 3 days after the corneal insult [32]. Since we had previously shown that the expression of CD11b was related to the surgical trauma of lenticule extraction, the difference in the results between the two studies may be explained by differences in surgical technique in lenticule extraction. The expression of fibronectin appeared around the incision as well as along the anterior and posterior extracted lenticule planes at day 1 postoperatively (Figs. 2.5a and 2.5b), and the staining intensity in these two sites increased at week 1 postoperatively (Figs. 2.5c and 2.5d). Studies on rabbit wound-healing models have shown that 1 day after an incision on the cornea, fibronectin appeared at the site of injury. During the following 1–2 weeks, the increased fibronectin provided a provisional matrix to support the

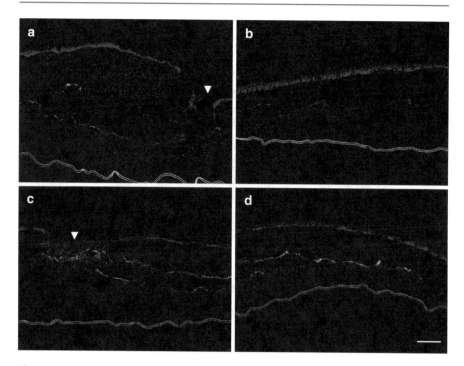

Fig. 2.5 Immunohistochemical staining showing the expression of fibronectin in rabbit corneas 1 day (**a, b**) and 1 week (**c, d**) at the incision (**a, c**; *arrowheads*) and extracted lenticule plane (**b, d**) after −4.0 D SMILE. The expression of fibronectin appeared around the incision as well as extracted lenticule plane at day 1 (**a, b**), and the staining intensity in these two sites became greater at week 1 postoperatively (**c, d**). Original magnification: 200×, scale bar 100 μm

migration of the remaining epithelial cells or keratocytes to cover the area of the defect [33, 34]. After 2 weeks, the wound-healing response was complete, and the expression of fibronectin began to decrease [33]. This explains why the expression of fibronectin appeared more distinct around both the small vertical incision and extracted lenticule plane at week 1 after SMILE. Heat shock protein 47 (HSP47) is a stress protein and functions as a collagen-specific molecular chaperon. It is induced in response to stress applied to cells [35, 36]. Unlike the staining pattern of CD11b that mainly appeared in the vertical incision and resolved at 1 week following SMILE, the expression of HSP47 was observed throughout the whole cornea at day 1 postoperatively (Figs. 2.6a, b), suggesting that the laser-induced cell stress may affect the whole layer of cornea, as well as the small incision site. The HSP47-positive cells significantly reduced at 1 week postoperatively (Figs. 2.6c, d).

Corneal backscatter light intensity (LI) depth graphics (Z-scan), a feature of in vivo confocal microscopy (IVCM), has been reported to be used to evaluate corneal stromal reaction, keratocyte activation, and objective haze grading after refractive surgery [37–39]. Our group has also used IVCM to evaluate and compare the early corneal wound healing and inflammatory response after Fs-LASIK and FLEx

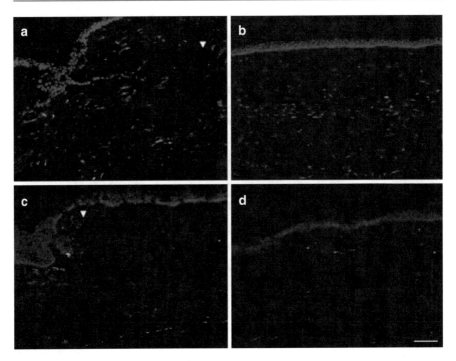

Fig. 2.6 Immunohistochemical staining showing the expression of HSP47 in rabbit corneas 1 day (**a**, **b**) and 1 week (**c**, **d**) at the incision (**a**, **c**; *arrowheads*) and extracted lenticule plane (**b**, **d**) after −4.0 D SMILE. HSP47-positive cells were observed throughout the whole cornea but significantly reduced at 1 week postoperatively. Original magnification: 200×, scale bar 100 μm

in a rabbit model by semi-quantifying the reflectivity level using ImageJ software [26]. The difference in reflectivity level between the two groups was only significant at higher refractive corrections (>6.0 D myopic correction), with higher reflectivity level in the Fs-LASIK group (Fig. 2.7). That was because greater levels of correction required more tissue to be ablated and longer exposure to the excimer, hence delivering more energy to the cornea. On the contrary, in the refractive lenticule extraction (ReLEx) procedure, either in FLEx or SMILE, the laser energy simply cuts a different shaped lenticule with an energy of only about 0.58 J (unpublished data were from Carl Zeiss Meditec), and the energy levels did not differ significantly between different attempted corrections [26].

There are other factors that also have an impact on the extent of corneal wound healing and inflammatory response after SMILE, including the laser cut energy level (laser cut energy index), spot size, and spacing setting [40]. These parameters should be taken into account when interpreting the wound-healing results among different studies.

Although SMILE has been reported as a safe and efficient strategy to treat a wide range of myopia [41], and the energy levels to cut different-thickness lenticules do

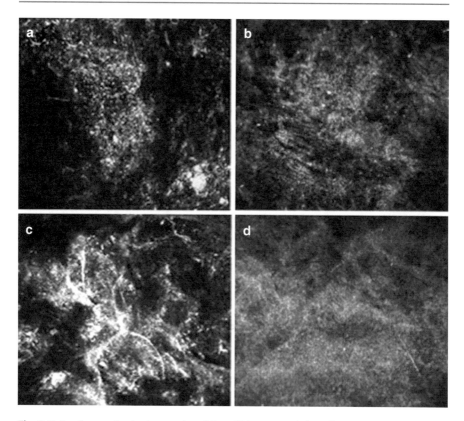

Fig. 2.7 In vivo confocal micrographs of the rabbit corneas 1 day after −3.0 D Fs-LASIK (**a**), −3.0 D SMILE (**b**), −9.0 D Fs-LASIK (**c**), and −9.0 D SMILE (**d**), at the flap interface (Fs-LASIK) or cap interface (SMILE). The interface site was acellular and light reflective. The difference in reflectivity level between two groups was only significant at higher corrections (**c**, **d**), with higher reflectivity level in the Fs-LASIK group

not differ significantly between different attempted corrections, the differences in the ease of dissection and lenticule extraction among different power of corrections may still have an impact on the postoperative wound-healing and inflammatory response. In low myopic treatment, the delineation and dissection of the anterior surface of the lenticule may be difficult because the lenticule is thin. When the initial dissection undermines the posterior surface of the lenticule, the surgery may become difficult, as the lenticule sticks to the anterior corneal cap and is difficult to be extracted [42]. Furthermore, it is more challenging to extract the lenticule when doing low myopic treatment because the lenticule is thin. These increased manipulations may lead to a greater extent of inflammatory process. A study to evaluate the wound healing and inflammatory response following different power of SMILE corrections is ongoing in our institute.

2.2.2 Clinical Study

The sequelae of corneal wound healing in refractive surgery can lead to undesirable complications, such as corneal haze, epithelial ingrowth, and regression [6, 11–13, 43, 44]. In a large study evaluating more than 1,500 SMILE procedures [31], the authors reported that trace corneal haze (grade 0.5–1) was the most frequent postoperative complication noted 3 months after SMILE (127/1,574 eyes, 8.1 %). Among these 127 eyes that had corneal haze, 10 of them had notes of perioperative complications, with six cases of difficult lenticule extraction and four minor tears at the incision. These perioperative complications may trigger greater extent of inflammatory cytokines release, leading to corneal haze. In 10 eyes (10/1,574 eyes, 0.6 %), a few islands of epithelial cells were seen near the incision site, and this epithelial ingrowth disappeared spontaneously after approximately 1 year postoperatively in 5 of the eyes. In five cases (0.3 %), the patients presented with one or more interface infiltrates 1 week after surgery. Samples were taken for microbiological investigation, but specific pathogens could not be identified. Four eyes (0.3 %) experienced interface inflammation during the first week after surgery and were successfully treated with dexamethasone eye drops.

Agca et al. [45] conducted a randomized clinical trial enrolling 30 patients who underwent SMILE in one eye and Fs-LASIK in the fellow eye and reported that the mean backscattered LI at all measured depths were significantly higher in the SMILE group than the Fs-LASIK group at all postoperative visits from 1 week to 3 months. The authors stated that this increased corneal backscatter in the early postoperative period in the SMILE group did not necessarily result in decreased vision, increased incidence of complications, or increased inflammation, but it reflected a different healing response after SMILE, and whether this difference has any positive or negative clinical consequences is still unknown

Kamiya et al. [46] also reported that transient interface haze was the most common adverse complication in SMILE, although it was mild and resolved with time. The authors also stated that this mild degree of interface haze may account for the tendency for a slight delay of visual recovery in the early postoperative period (especially 1 week postoperatively) in SMILE or FLEx compared to Fs-LASIK.

Topical steroid treatment has been used in limiting corneal haze and myopic regression in highly myopic patients after photorefractive keratectomy (PRK) [47]. For LASIK patients, it was reported in a large clinical study that topical steroids significantly decreased the incidence of corneal haze at week 1 but was associated with decreased stability of refraction in more highly myopic eyes [48]. Likewise, although no large-scale and long-term follow-up data looking at the myopic regression after SMILE is available currently, topical steroids may not provide a beneficial role in preventing regression after SMILE, as the firing laser type, laser energy, and resultant inflammatory response in SMILE is more similar to LASIK and different from PRK. At present, there is no standard protocol for topical steroids use following SMILE. Most of the institutes, including our institute, use a regimen of topical steroids four times a day for 1 week with a tapering dose for the following week [31, 41, 49]. Some institutes use postoperative steroids for even shorter period [50]. However, in cases of difficult lenticule extractions, higher-dose steroids maybe required if extensive manipulations occurs at the incision site.

Conclusions

Corneal wound-healing process has a major impact on the postoperative visual outcomes, complications, and corneal biomechanical changes after ReLEx®. As ReLEx is a newly arisen technique, there are only a few studies in the literature reporting its wound healing and inflammatory response at present. Based on rabbit SMILE models, SMILE leaves a small epithelial incision that heals within 1 week. The extracted lenticule plane itself and the remaining stromal bed undergo little inflammatory response, and the inflammatory response seems to primarily result from surgical manipulation to extract the lenticule, rather than laser itself. The postoperative complications resulting from impaired wound healing or inflammatory response, such as corneal haze or epithelial ingrowth, are reported to be low and were mainly associated with perioperative complications, such as difficult lenticule extraction. However, more large-scale, long-term follow-up clinical studies are required.

References

1. Buratto L, Slade SG, Tavolato M (2012) Chap 4: LASIK: the evolution of refractive surgery. SLACK Incorporated, Thorofare, p 37
2. Sugar A (2002) Ultrafast (femtosecond) laser refractive surgery. Curr Opin Ophthalmol 13(4):246–249
3. Vogel A, Schweiger P, Freiser A et al (1990) Intraocular Nd:YAG laser surgery: light-tissue interactions, damage range, and reduction of collateral effects. IEEE J Quantum Electron 26:2240–2260
4. Pepose JS (2008) Comparing femtosecond lasers. Cataract Refract Surg Today 45–51
5. Lubatschowski H (2008) Overview of commercially available femtosecond lasers in refractive surgery. J Refract Surg 24:S102–S107
6. Santhiago MR, Wilson SE (2012) Cellular effects after laser in situ keratomileusis flap formation with femtosecond lasers: a review. Cornea 31(2):198–205
7. de Paula FH, Khairallah CG, Niziol LM, Musch DC, Shtein RM (2012) Diffuse lamellar keratitis after laser in situ keratomileusis with femtosecond laser flap creation. J Cataract Refract Surg 38:1014–1019
8. Stonecipher KG, Dishler JG, Ignacio TS, Binder PS (2006) Transient light sensitivity after femtosecond laser flap creation: clinical findings and management. J Cataract Refract Surg 32:91–94
9. Azar DT, Chang JH, Han KY (2012) Wound healing after keratorefractive surgery: review of biological and optical considerations. Cornea 31(Suppl 1):S9–S19
10. Dupps WJ Jr, Wilson SE (2006) Biomechanics and wound healing in the cornea. Exp Eye Res 83(4):709–720
11. Vaddavalli PK, Hurmeric V, Wang J, Yoo SH (2012) Corneal haze following disruption of epithelial basement membrane on ultra-high-resolution OCT following femtosecond LASIK. J Refract Surg 28(1):72–74
12. Kanellopoulos AJ, Asimellis G (2014) Epithelial remodeling after femtosecond laser-assisted high myopic LASIK: comparison of stand-alone with LASIK combined with prophylactic high-fluence cross-linking. Cornea 33(5):463–469

13. Vaddavalli PK, Yoo SH (2011) Femtosecond laser in-situ keratomileusis flap configurations. Curr Opin Ophthalmol 22(4):245–250
14. Mohan RR, Mohan RR, Kim WJ, Wilson SE (2000) Modulation of TNF-alpha-induced apoptosis in corneal fibroblasts by transcription factor NF-kb. Invest Ophthalmol Vis Sci 41:1327–1336
15. Tuominen IS, Tervo TM, Teppo AM et al (2001) Human tear fluid PDGF-BB, TNF-alpha and TGF-beta1 vs corneal haze and regeneration of corneal epithelium and subbasal nerve plexus after PRK. Exp Eye Res 72:631–641
16. Mohan RR, Mohan RR, Kim WJ et al (2000) Modulation of TNF-alpha induced apoptosis in corneal fibroblasts by transcription factor NF-kb. Invest Ophthalmol Vis Sci 41:1327–1334
17. Mohan RR, Liang Q, Kim WJ, Helena MC, Baerveldt F, Wilson SE (1997) Apoptosis in the cornea: further characterization of Fas/Fas ligand system. Exp Eye Res 65:575–589
18. Jester JV, Moller-Pedersen T, Huang J, Sax CM, Kays WT, Cavangh HD, Petroll WM, Piatigorsky J (1999) The cellular basis of corneal transparency: evidence for 'corneal crystallins'. J Cell Sci 112:613–622
19. Jester JV, Petroll WM, Cavanagh HD (1999) Corneal stromal wound healing in refractive surgery: the role of myofibroblasts. Prog Retin Eye Res 18(3):311–356
20. Netto MV, Mohan RR, Sinha S, Sharma A, Dupps W, Wilson SE (2006) Stromal haze, myofibroblasts, and surface irregularity after PRK. Exp Eye Res 82:788–e797
21. Saika S (2004) TGF-beta signal transduction in corneal wound healing as a therapeutic target. Cornea 23:S25–S30
22. Torricelli AA, Wilson SE (2014) Cellular and extracellular matrix modulation of corneal stromal opacity. Exp Eye Res 129:151–60, pii: S0014-4835(14)00263-2
23. Ambati BK, Nozaki M, Singh N, Takeda A, Jani PD, Suthar T, Albuquerque RJ, Richter E, Sakurai E, Newcomb MT, Kleinman ME, Caldwell RB, Lin Q, Ogura Y, Orecchia A, Samuelson DA, Agnew DW, St Leger J, Green WR, Mahasreshti PJ, Curiel DT, Kwan D, Marsh H, Ikeda S, Leiper LJ, Collinson JM, Bogdanovich S, Khurana TS, Shibuya M, Baldwin ME, Ferrara N, Gerber HP, De Falco S, Witta J, Baffi JZ, Raisler BJ, Ambati J (2006) Corneal avascularity is due to soluble VEGF receptor-1. Nature 443(7114):993–997
24. Chang JH, Gabison EE, Kato T, Azar DT (2001) Corneal neovascularization. Curr Opin Ophthalmol 12(4):242–249
25. Tombran-Tink J, Chader GG, Johnson LV (1991) PEDF: a pigment epithelium-derived factor with potent neuronal differentiative activity. Exp Eye Res 53(3):411–414
26. Riau AK, Angunawela RI, Chaurasia SS, Lee WS, Tan DT, Mehta JS (2011) Early corneal wound healing and inflammatory responses after refractive lenticule extraction (ReLEx). Invest Ophthalmol Vis Sci 52(9):6213–6221
27. Nakamura M, Sato N, Chikama T, Hasegawa Y, Nishida T (1997) Fibronectin facilitates corneal epithelial wound healing in diabetic rats. Exp Eye Res 64(3):355–359
28. Dong Z, Zhou X, Wu J, Zhang Z, Li T, Zhou Z, Zhang S, Li G (2014) Small incision lenticule extraction (SMILE) and femtosecond laser LASIK: comparison of corneal wound healing and inflammation. Br J Ophthalmol 98(2):263–269
29. Kim WJ, Mohan RR, Mohan RR, Wilson SE (1999) Effect of PDGF, IL-1 alpha, and BMP2/4 on corneal fibroblast chemotaxis: expression of the platelet-derived growth factor system in the cornea. Invest Ophthalmol Vis Sci 40:1364–1372
30. Zieske JD, Mason VS, Wasson ME et al (1994) Basement membrane assembly and differentiation of cultured corneal cells: importance of culture environment and endothelial cell interaction. Exp Eye Res 214:621–633
31. Ivarsen A, Asp S, Hjortdal J (2014) Safety and complications of more than 1500 small-incision lenticule extraction procedures. Ophthalmology 121:822–828
32. Dartt DA, Bex P, D'Amore P (2011) Chapter 2: Sturucture and function of the tear film, ocular adnexa, cornea and conjunctiva in health and pathogenesis in disease. In: Ocular periphery and disorders, p 266
33. Nishida T (2012) The role of fibronectin in corneal wound healing explored by a physician-scientist. Jpn J Ophthalmol 56(5):417–431

34. Tervo K, van Setten GB, Beuerman RW, Virtanen I, Tarkkanen A, Tervo T (1991) Expression of tenascin and cellular fibronectin in the rabbit cornea after anterior keratectomy. Immunohistochemical study of wound healing dynamics. Invest Ophthalmol Vis Sci 32(11):2912–2918
35. Satoh M, Hirayoshi K, Yokota S, Hosokawa N, Nagata K (1996) Intracellular interaction of collagen-specific stress protein HSP47 with newly synthesized procollagen. J Cell Biol 133:469–483
36. Nagata K (1998) Expression and function of heat shock protein 47: a collagen-specific molecular chaperone in the endoplasmic reticulum. Matrix Biol 16(7):379–386
37. Møller-Pedersen T, Vogel M, Li HF, Petroll WM, Cavanagh HD, Jester JV (1997) Quantification of stro- mal thinning, epithelial thickness, and corneal haze after pho- torefractive keratectomy using in vivo confocal microscopy. Ophthalmology 104(3):360–368
38. Marchini G, Mastropasqua L, Pedrotti E, Nubile M, Ciancaglini M, Sbabo A (2006) Deep lamellar keratoplasty by intracorneal dissection: a prospective clinical and confocal microscopic study. Ophthalmology 113(8):1289–1300
39. Prasher P, Muftuoglu O, Bowman RW et al (2009) Tandem scanning confocal microscopy of cornea after descemet stripping automated endothelial keratoplasty. Eye Contact Lens 35(4):196–202
40. Hu MY, McCulley JP, Cavanagh HD, Bowman RW, Verity SM, Mootha VV, Petroll WM (2007) Comparison of the corneal response to laser in situ keratomileusis with flap creation using the FS15 and FS30 femtosecond lasers: clinical and confocal microscopy findings. J Cataract Refract Surg 33(4):673–681
41. Vestergaard A, Ivarsen AR, Asp S, Hjortdal JØ (2012) Small-incision lenticule extraction for moderate to high myopia: predictability, safety, and patient satisfaction. J Cataract Refract Surg 38(11):2003–2010
42. Liu YC, Pujara T, Mehta JS (2014) New instruments for lenticule extraction in small incision lenticule extraction (SMILE). PLoS One 9(12), e113774
43. Farah SG, Azar DT, Gurdal C et al (1998) Laser in situ keratomileusis: literature review of a developing technique. J Cataract Refract Surg 24:989–1006
44. Hersh PS, Brint SF, Maloney RK et al (1998) Photorefractive keratectomy versus laser in situ keratomileusis for moderate to high myopia. Ophthalmology 105:1512–1523
45. Agca A, Ozgurhan EB, Yildirim Y, Cankaya KI, Guleryuz NB, Alkin Z, Ozkaya A, Demirok A, Yilmaz OF (2014) Corneal backscatter analysis by in vivo confocal microscopy: fellow eye comparison of small incision lenticule extraction and femtosecond laser-assisted LASIK. J Ophthalmol 2014:265012. doi:10.1155/2014/265012
46. Kamiya K, Shimizu K, Igarashi A, Kobashi H (2014) Visual and refractive outcomes of femtosecond lenticule extraction and small-incision lenticule extraction for myopia. Am J Ophthalmol 157(1):128–134.e2
47. Vetrugno M, Maino A, Quaranta GM, Cardia L (2001) The effect of early steroid treatment after PRK on clinical and refractive outcomes. Acta Ophthalmol Scand 79(1):23–27
48. Price FW Jr, Willes L, Price M, Lyng A, Ries J (2001) A prospective, randomized comparison of the use versus non-use of topical corticosteroids after laser in situ keratomileusis. Ophthalmology 108(7):1236–1244
49. Vestergaard AH, Grauslund J, Ivarsen AR, Hjortdal JØ (2014) Efficacy, safety, predictability, contrast sensitivity, and aberrations after femtosecond laser lenticule extraction. J Cataract Refract Surg 40(3):403–11
50. Sekundo W, Kunert KS, Blum M (2011) Small incision corneal refractive surgery using the small incision lenticule extraction (SMILE) procedure for the correction of myopia and myopic astigmatism: results of a 6 month prospective study. Br J Ophthalmol 95(3):335–339

Corneal Nerve and Keratocyte Response to ReLEx® Surgery

3

Leonardo Mastropasqua and Mario Nubile

Contents

3.1   Introduction

Corneal laser refractive surgery gained popularity among ophthalmologists since the beginning of the 1990s of the last century and rapidly substituted the old manual incisional surgery such as radial and astigmatic keratotomies [1–3]. In fact, excimer laser surgical procedures for the treatment of ametropias changed completely the

L. Mastropasqua, MD (✉) • M. Nubile, MD
Ophthalmology Clinic, Center for Excellence in Ophthalmology, National High-Tech Eye Center, University of Chieti, Pescara, Italy
e-mail: mastropa@unich.it; mnubile@unich.it

© Springer International Publishing Switzerland 2015
W. Sekundo (ed.), *Small Incision Lenticule Extraction (SMILE):*
Principles, Techniques, Complication Management, and Future Concepts,
DOI 10.1007/978-3-319-18530-9_3

approach to refractive corrections, basing the modification of the corneal shape on the mechanism of the so-called laser "photoablation" of the corneal stroma, which makes possible to sculpt the cornea with microscopic accuracy [4]. Laser in situ keratomileusis (LASIK), photorefractive keratectomy (PRK), and, among the surface ablation procedures, the variations called laser-assisted subepithelial keratectomy (LASEK) and Epi-LASIK represented the most exploited, successfully used and evolving corneal laser surgical interventions for the correction of myopia and other ametropias [5, 6].

Despite the great precision of corneal refractive excimer laser ablations and the recent improvement of the techniques, drawbacks intrinsic to the procedures still persist unsolved, including surgical induced nerve damages and triggering of stromal wound healing and keratocytes changes [7]. These postsurgical corneal alterations are generally transient but in some cases may be persistent and often can lead to undesirable side effects and symptoms in treated patients. Damage to the corneal nerve plexus is frequent cause of corneal neurotrophic epitheliopathy, with related dry eye symptoms and altered tear film dynamics, while keratocyte apoptosis, stromal inflammation and wound healing can be responsible for regression of the achieved corrections and loss of corneal transparency (haze) [7].

Recent investigations suggest that ReLEx techniques, due to the photodisruption mechanism and the flap-less approach (for SMILE), may exert different effects on corneal nerve fibers and keratocytes after myopic and astigmatic refractive correction as compared to the traditional excimer laser-based surface ablation and LASIK techniques. The aim of this chapter is to provide a description of the in vivo findings of corneal nerve and keratocyte response to ReLEx surgery and to discuss the pathophysiology of these changes along with the potential for clinical advantages and future development.

3.2 Surgical Anatomy of the Corneal Nerves and of the Stromal Keratocytes

3.2.1 Nerve Fibers

The cornea is a highly sensitive structure and is innervated by the ophthalmic division of the trigeminal nerve. Superficial corneal nerve density is estimated to be approximately 300–600 times that of skin and 20 times that of tooth pulp [8]. The human cornea receives most of its sensory innervation from the two long ciliary nerves that enter the posterior globe adjacent to the optic nerve and course forward in the suprachoroidal space at the nasal and temporal meridians [9]. Prior to reaching the corneoscleral limbus, the nerves branch into smaller bundles and anastomose repetitively with branches of the short ciliary nerves that approach the limbus radially from all directions. The nerves that enter the cornea can be considered as mixed sensory and autonomic nerves. Recent investigations redefined the knowledge of the neural architecture and distribution of the corneal nerves [10–12].

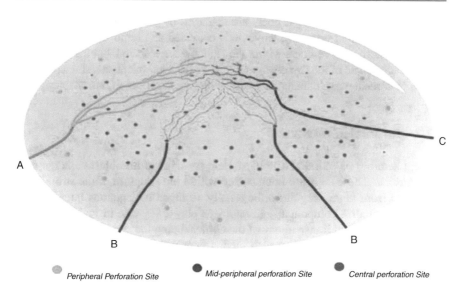

Peripheral Perforation Site   Mid-peripheral perforation Site   Central perforation Site

Fig. 3.1 Schematic representation of the anatomy of corneal nerves. Nerve fibers enter the cornea at the limbal region and then run radially toward the center as stromal fibers. These fibers tend to reach the stromal superficial layers and perforate the Bowman's layer at different topographical locations (*different colors*). The sites of Bowman's membrane perforation are depicted by *colored dots*. After gaining the superficial location, they give origin to the subbasal fibers

Approximately 30–60 thick nerve bundles enter the human cornea in a relatively equal distribution around the circumference of the limbus and thereafter run toward the central cornea, dividing into several branches in the peripheral area. In the stroma, nerves organize in parallel to collagen lamellae, branch into smaller fascicles as they become more superficial and form interconnections (anterior stromal plexus). It is evident that nerve density increases, while nerve diameter thins moving anteriorly toward the superficial stroma. It is remarkable to note that a small number of stromal nerves terminate as free endings, while some fibers directly innervate keratocytes [13]. After passing through the Bowman's zone, the original stromal fibers terminate into "bulb-like thickenings" from which multiple subbasal nerve arise [10]. The stromal nerves penetrate the Bowman's layer (perforation sites) mainly in the mid-peripheral cornea with relatively fewer perforation sites in the central or peripheral cornea (See Fig. 3.1). Approximately 25–30 perforation sites were observed in the human central cornea versus 125–160 perforation sites in the mid-peripheral cornea [10]. After the perforation nerve fibers branch and divide further and then run below the epithelium to originate the subbasal plexus.

It is of interest to consider that when surface refractive ablations (i.e., PRK) are performed, the epithelial removal and the superficial ablation remove the central Bowman's layer and anterior stroma, therefore eliminating the epithelial, subbasal, and most anterior stromal nerve fibers. In case of LASIK surgery, although the epithelium, Bowman's zone, and very anterior stroma are preserved from ablation in the flap, the nerve fibers are resected peripherally due to the flap circumferential side cut, while deeper stromal fibers are damaged by the ablation under the flap. When a femtosecond refractive lenticule is dissected and removed, in the SMILE technique, stromal nerve fibers within the lenticule are resected, but the absence of surface damage and of the flap creation represent the anatomical basis for a different pattern of corneal nerve damage that will be discussed further in this chapter.

3.2.2   Stromal Keratocytes

Corneal keratocytes (corneal fibroblasts) are specialized fibroblast cells residing in the stroma. These cells are interspersed within the structure of the stroma that is built up from highly regular orthogonally arranged collagenous lamellae and extracellular matrix components. Keratocytes play a key role in maintaining the stromal structure and transparency of the cornea, being the source of stromal collagen and proteoglycans. They also mediate corneal wound healing and tissue repair and are capable of undergoing phenotypic transformations in wounds due to the influence of growth factors and cytokines. These specialized cells are therefore involved in healing corneal wounds and synthesizing its components. In the unperturbed cornea, keratocytes are normally quiescent, but they can rapidly respond and change into repair phenotypes following injury [14, 15]. Stromal keratocyte density has been evaluated both ex vivo and in vivo, and it is known to be higher in the anterior third of the stroma, while it progressively decreases in the mid and rear stroma (Fig. 3.2).

In excimer laser surface ablation techniques, the very anterior keratocytes (depending on the ablation depth) are damaged, and apoptosis mechanisms, with subsequent wound healing cascade, are triggered in the most keratocyte-populated area of the stroma. In LASIK technique the keratocyte and stromal healing phenomena occur at a deeper level (in the residual stromal bed under the flap-stroma and the ablated tissue), where the keratocyte density is lower. In SMILE and to some extent in FLEx techniques, the unique use of femtosecond laser dissection with no photoablation induces a different pattern, of keratocyte changes and wound healing (in the anterior-mid stroma), characterized by less apoptosis and inflammation, as already discussed in the previous chapter.

3.2.3   In Vivo Confocal Microscopy of the Cornea: An Imaging Technique for Nerves and Keratocytes

In vivo confocal microscopy (IVCM) has gained a notable popularity and consensus as a powerful imaging tool among cornea specialists in the last two decades. It is a noninvasive diagnostic imaging system that allows viewing of tissues, in particular the cornea at its microscopic details, one depth level at a time [16–19]. This kind of microscopes is designed for noninvasive, real-time, in vivo examination of tissues without the need of stains or dyes but does require operator-dependent expertise and skill in optimizing the quality of the obtained images and their interpretation.

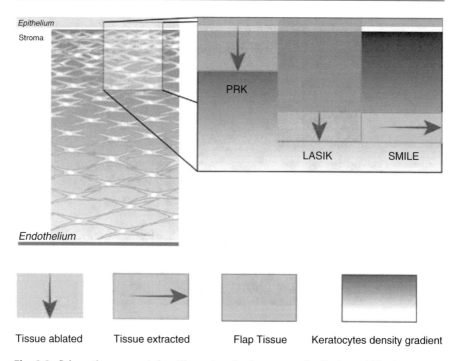

Fig. 3.2 Schematic representation illustrating the keratocyte distribution within the corneal stroma and the surgical anatomy of three different corneal refractive surgical techniques: PRK, LASIK, and SMILE (section)

Currently two different confocal technologies are available for clinical use: the laser scanning and the white-light scanning confocal microscopy. These two confocal systems clearly differ in the capacity of ocular tissue imaging depending on the type of light source used. White-light confocal microscopy offers a detailed view of the corneal layers, provides an optical pachymetry of the entire cornea or of selected sublayers, and allows for automatic cell counts (i.e., keratocytes and endothelial cell density), but the imaging quality is affected by tissue transparency and stromal edema more than laser scanning confocal systems. Due to the fact that the cornea is generally a nearly transparent tissue, with minimal light absorption, the increase in axial resolution allows confocal microscopy to scan optical sections of the entire corneal thickness producing high magnification (between 600 and 1,000×) "en face images" of the cornea (maintaining lateral and axial resolution within values comprised between 1 and 3 µm and 5 up to 10 µm, respectively). Almost all anatomical corneal layers are clearly imaged by confocal microscopy: superficial epithelium, basal epithelium, Bowman's membrane, subepithelial nerve plexus, corneal stroma with resident keratocytes, deep nerve fibers, Descemet's membrane, and endothelium. Figure 3.3 presents a composition of images illustrating confocal microscopic anatomy of the central human corneal layers. As visible in the figure, in vivo confocal images are oriented parallel to the microscope objective and to the corneal

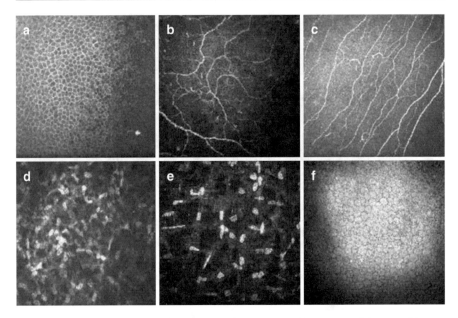

Fig. 3.3 Composition of images illustrating confocal microscopic anatomy of the central human corneal layers, with emphasis on visualizing nerve fibers and keratocytes. (**a**) Basal epithelium. (**b**, **c**) Different pattern of subepithelial nerve plexus. (**d**) High density of anterior stromal kerato-cytes. (**e**) Mid-stromal keratocytes present a lower density. (**f**) Normal endothelial cell mosaic

surface, differently than histological specimens, which are sectioned perpendicular to the surface of the cornea, and thus the observer has to become familiar with the imaging in the coronal plane.

3.3 Nerve Fibers Change After ReLEx Refractive Surgery: Morphology and Clinical Meaning

3.3.1 Nerve Fibers and Tear Film Alterations After Excimer Laser Surgery

Any kind of subtractive laser refractive surgery has the disadvantages of inducing a variable degree of damage to the corneal nerve fibers. It is well known that the integrity of nerve fibers is fundamental for the physiological maintenance of the ocular surface tear film dynamics and corneal epithelial homeostasis. Tear secretion is regulated through a neural reflex initiated by trigeminal primary afferent neurons innervating the corneal epithelium. Dry eye phenomena may be induced by a dysfunction in the tear-secreting glands or in the neuronal circuit regulating these glands [20].

Patients' complain of dry eye symptoms and related epitheliopathy commonly occur after traditional refractive surgery techniques. The most frequently reported manifestations are ocular dryness that takes place in almost 40 % of LASIK (laser-assisted in situ keratomileusis) and PRK (photorefractive keratectomy) treated eyes, but also nonspecific ocular surface discomfort associated with mild corneal epitheliopathy and reduced lubrication may occur [21]. At the present time LASIK (either performed with microkeratomes or with Fs-Laser) is considered as one of the gold standard refractive procedures, supported by numerous investigations, for its visual outcomes and rapid postoperative recovery. The LASIK technique induces morphological and functional effects on the corneal surface. Changes in corneal shape, tear film dynamic, and subepithelial innervation after surgery exert a significant influence in ocular discomfort syndrome onset. The impact of these factors produces detrimental effects to visual results including fluctuation of vision quality and decrease of contrast sensitivity and, in some cases, of best spectacle-corrected visual acuity [22]. One of the key points to consider in the occurrence of these phenomena is the fact that different patients may present a variable spectrum of symptoms to identical surgical stimuli and that preexisting dry eye before surgery can be a risk factor for severe ocular discomfort after refractive surgery.

As explained, excimer laser-based procedures (either LASIK or surface ablation techniques such as PRK) result in a sudden central corneal nerve fiber damage related to the flap cut, in LASIK, and to the excimer photoablation of the anterior stroma containing nerve fibers, that takes time to recover, often only partially. The wound healing of central corneal subepithelial nerve fibers has been reported to be only slightly different between LASIK and similar flap-based procedures, regarding the time-to-recovery and the morphological appearance of the regenerated nerve plexus. At 1 month after surgery, the central cornea appears devoid of nerve fibers in conventional LASIK procedure, sub-Bowman's keratomileusis (SBK), and femtosecond laser-assisted LASIK (Fs-LASIK) [23]. The process of reinnervation begins in the early period after surgery in the peripheral flap region with the formation of thin non-branching fibers crossing the side cut. Nerve morphology changes rapidly across the following months reaching the central 3 mm area at 6 month [23]. In spite of this nerve regrowth, the density and the nerve morphology remain altered for years after surgery, representing the basis for some clinical conditions of dryness and recurrent superficial epithelial punctate erosions. Surface excimer laser ablations showed a faster recovery time, with 2 year of mean time-to-restoration against 5 year of the flap-based procedures [24].

Along with the corneal neural impairment, patients show an altered corneal sensitivity that follows a similar pattern by decreasing significantly immediately after, persisting reduced in the first 3 months, and returning to normal values at 6 months after surgery [25]. Previous investigations reported a persistent noncomplete normalization at 1 year and more [26].

The risk of developing "dry eye syndrome" appears to be correlated with the degree of preoperative myopia and the depth of laser ablation/stromal dissection; moreover, in dry eye-affected patients, the risk of myopic regression is increased [27, 28]. The status of the ocular surface and tear film before and after refractive surgery can adversely affect the outcomes in terms of complications, refractive results, optical quality, patient satisfaction, and the severity and duration of dry eye after LASIK [29].

Recently femtosecond laser systems became available for the clinical use in corneal refractive surgery and favored improvements in the reliability of LASIK procedures by increasing flap precision (thickness, shape, diameter), setting up planar configuration of the flap cut geometry, and giving more predictable depth of dissection and reduction of intraoperative complications incidence [30]. Despite these advantages with Fs-laser-created flaps, corneal nerve plexus presents the above-described modification and remains affected by severe damage for a long time. In fact, the flap creation implies the transection of all nerve fibers at the lamellar border. In spite of the better alignment of flap margins achieved with Fs-LASIK, the reinnervation process emerges to be similar to the well-known microkeratome-LASIK procedures. Central nerve fibers density reduction and slow progressive recovery turned out to be comparable in both techniques as long as 3 years after surgery [30]. Similarly, the incidence of dry eye symptoms after surgery is similar in both procedures. Therefore, the planar configuration of thin Fs-LASIK flaps is not associated with faster reinnervation compared with the microkeratome flaps and does not provide clinically significant advantages in terms of induced neurotrophic epitheliopathy. Patients complaining of post-refractive surgery dry eye symptoms are generally treated by frequent instillations of lubricant eye drops and occasionally local steroids and/or topical cyclosporin A for weeks to months after surgery; however, there is no recognized and definite treatment for such condition.

3.3.2 Corneal Nerve Fibers After ReLEx: Anatomical Bases and Scientific Evidence

Femtosecond laser refractive surgery received a notable advancement with the introduction of "all-femto" SMILE technique. The capacity of the femtosecond laser of designing intrastromal dissection planes with three-dimensional cut complex geometry helps the surgeons to remove corneal tissue without a flap by creating a lenticule and a small incision to extract it. The first dissection plane designs the backside face of the lenticule, while the second one creates its anterior face and extends further to form a spaced intrastromal pocket to facilitate the extraction maneuvers (edge of the so-called cap). The complete procedure happens without affecting the superficial tissue, fashioning an intrastromal "disk" that can be easily extracted through the 40–50 arc degrees single superficial incision.

The basis that explains the pattern of nerve fiber resection induced by SMILE (similar to other refractive surgical procedure) relies in the anatomy of the intracorneal distribution of the fibers that give origin to the subbasal nerve plexus and of the topography of emerging fibers that penetrate the Bowman's layer (BL) running, thereafter, superficially. As explained previously in this chapter, the stromal nerves, coming from the suprachoroidal space through the limbal region, course toward the center in a radial manner and penetrate the Bowman's layer at different locations, mostly situated in the mid-peripheral zone (outside the central 6 mm), creating, thereafter, the subbasal plexus. A schematic representation illustrating the nerve fiber pathway that runs centripetally is presented in Figs. 3.1 and 3.4a. When

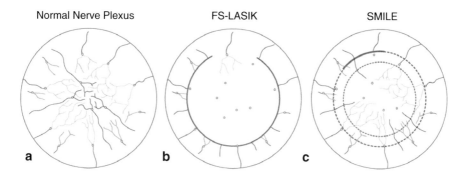

Normal Nerve Plexus   FS-LASIK   SMILE

Fig. 3.4 (**a**) Stromal nerve fiber bundles run centripetally and toward the surface perforating the Bowman's layer (spots indicated by *yellow circles*). Once the fibers penetrate the BL, the subbasal nerve plexus is originated. *Different colors* illustrate the subbasal fibers originating from central (*red*), paracentral (*light blue*), and peripheral (*green*) perforating stromal fibers, respectively. (**b**) In the LASIK procedure, all fibers are cut throughout the extension of the 300–310° degree of arc flap side cut; moreover all deeper fibers are disrupted within the photoablation area. (**c**) With the SMILE procedure, in the absence of a full flap side cut, peripheral nerve fibers are resected only were the 50° arc of the incision is placed (*thick red line*). Moreover fibers are resected if rising superficially to perforate the BL within the area of the created and extracted refractive lenticule. The other fibers that had penetrated the BL outside the lenticule area may run undisturbed as subbasal nerve plexus (for simplicity, central subbasal surviving fibers are not depicted in the central zone)

a flap-based technique (LASIK, Fs-LASIK, or FLEx) is performed, all nerve fibers that are running across the flap side-cut circumference are resected (the majority of the central and paracentral stromal fibers). The excimer laser ablation on the stromal bed further vaporizes remaining deeper stromal fibers. Only the fibers that run in the region of the flap hinge (few fibers) may course undisturbed within the lifted flap as subbasal fibers (see Fig. 3.4b). This supposed mechanism is in agreement with the described clinical and confocal observations that reported a remarkable reduction of corneal sensitivity and of the central subbasal corneal nerve plexus after LASIK.

On the other hand, when a SMILE procedure is performed, it is presumed that a different pattern of nerve resection occurs:

1. A certain amount of fibers running centripetally in the superficial stroma and in the subepithelial zone are resected due to the side cut where the incision is placed.
2. Other stromal fibers that run toward the surface perforating the Bowman's zone inside the refractive lenticule and cap area might be interrupted by the lenticule/cap planar dissection itself.
3. Conversely, fibers that gained the superficial subepithelial location after perforating the BL in areas located outside the lenticule/cap area may run untouched (inside the stromal and epithelial component of the cap) over the refractive zone without interruption with the exception of the mentioned peripheral incision (see Fig. 3.4c).

Some recent investigations have evaluated the corneal innervation and corneal sensitivity after ReLEx surgery. Authors that investigated changes in corneal sensitivity reported it to be significantly better after SMILE than after LASIK in every corneal area. Interestingly, corneal sensitivity values were found to reach preoperative levels as soon as 3 months after SMILE surgery, therefore suggesting that long-lasting changes, typical after LASIK procedures, should not occur after flap-less ReLEx SMILE surgery [31]. Vestergaard et al. evaluated corneal sensitivity and used confocal microscopy to study the subbasal nerve plexus morphology comparing two groups of femtosecond laser refractive surgery treated patients: the SMILE procedure as compared to the FLEx technique (the original approach to all-femto refractive myopic lenticule extraction, based on a complete flap lifting) [32]. The authors observed a better corneal sensitivity and a significantly higher density of central corneal nerve fibers as observed by confocal microscopy in the SMILE group with respect to the FLEx group at 6 months follow-up time. This study highlighted the importance of a flap-less procedure to favor a rapid nerve restoration; however, it does not take into account the early postoperative phase, and the LASIK technique was not investigated. Another investigation used in vivo confocal microscopy to evaluate changes of corneal innervation following SMILE surgery as compared to Fs-LASIK-treated eyes [33]. It reported a decrease in subbasal nerve fiber density less severe after SMILE in comparison to Fs-LASIK in the early postoperative phase (1 week to 3 months), while nerve density reached similar values at 6 months following both procedures. Nerve density values were found to correlate well with corneal aesthesiometry.

As explained, by the means of laser scanning in vivo confocal microscopy (IVCM), remarkable differences in the induced subbasal nerve fiber changes and subsequent nerve regeneration patterns can be found between flap-based refractive procedures (FS-LASIK and FLeX) and SMILE for similar myopic corrections.

When studying the peripheral nerve fiber integrity (in the areas corresponding to the flap side cut in the LASIK and the lenticule/cap area in the SMILE group, respectively), all fibers running centripetally are resected by the presence of the side cut. This concept is illustrated in (Fig. 3.4b), and confocal images are presented in Fig. 3.5. In flap-based procedures (Fs-LASIK or FLEx), the fibers are circumferentially interrupted by the flap side cut at the time of surgery. The following stromal excimer ablation (or lenticule removal in FLEx) further contributes to damage deeper fibers (Fig. 3.5a). In the SMILE procedure, peripheral fibers may be observed running centripetally, non-resected, in the area overlying the edge of the lenticular lamellar cut as shown in Fig. 3.5b. As it happens in LASIK, the superficial radial nerve fibers are resected where the SMILE incision is placed (Fig. 3.5c).

In LASIK treatments the inferred mechanisms responsible for corneal nerve damage include:

1. The peripheral transection of the nerve superficial nerve fibers that perforated the BL outside the flap area (flap side cut)
2. Resection of stromal nerve fibers crossing at any level the planar dissection of the flap
3. Further damage to deeper stromal fibers by the excimer photoablation

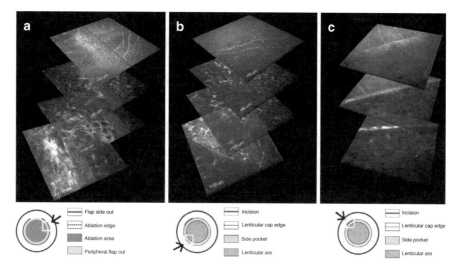

Fig. 3.5 Side-cut IVCM stack reconstruction. FS-LASIK (**a**), SMILE periphery (lenticule edge) (**b**), and SMILE incision (**c**). (**a**) In FSL-LASIK all fibers are resected throughout the extension (approximately 300°) of side cut of the flap (*top panel* shows resected fibers at the flap border 1 week after surgery; *underlying panels* show deeper stromal layers). (**b**) In SMILE non-damaged superficial fibers can be observed (*top panel*). They typically run over the lenticule stromal edge (*bottom panel*), toward the center, as they perforated the BL outside the lenticule-cap dissection. (**c**) The "small incision" represents a zone of superficial nerve fiber resection in the SMILE technique (*top panel*)

These features may explain the fact that, soon after surgery, the central nerve fibers density is markedly reduced in the LASIK treatments (Fig. 3.6a). The drop in central nerve fiber density produced by LASIK surgery is considered to be as high as 80–95 % [22–24, 30, 33, 34]. A partial recovery of the fiber density takes months to occur.

Conversely, in the SMILE technique, the reduction of the nerve fiber density was found to be significantly lower with faster central reinnervation than LASIK. Approximately 20–40 % of the central fibers are spared by SMILE surgery [31–34]. The reasons for partial nerve sparing in SMILE are:

1. Absence of the side cut that transects all edge-crossing fibers
2. Smaller area of the lenticule planar cut (6.5 mm in average plus the small pocket dissection) that is approximately 30 % smaller than LASIK flap cut [35]
3. Preservation of the integrity of the crossing fibers that reached the superficial subbasal location outside the lenticule-cap area (probably 20–30 %), as shown in (Fig. 3.5b)
4. Absence of excimer laser collateral stromal damage (further discussed in the last paragraph of this chapter)

These features probably play an important role in maintaining a partial corneal innervation in the early postoperative period and may be also responsible for the

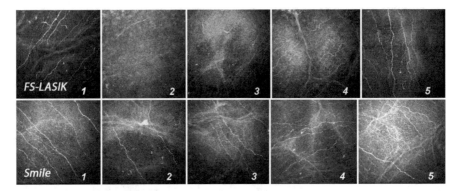

Fig. 3.6 In vivo confocal microscopy images of the central subbasal nerve plexus before and after FS-LASIK (*top line*) and SMILE (*bottom line*). *1* Preoperative, *2* 1 week, *3* 1 month, *4* 3 months, *5* 6 months. Note that distinct subbasal fibers are visible at 1 week and 1 month after SMILE surgery; recovery of nerve fiber density takes a longer time after LASIK

faster nerve regrowth observed in the first months after surgery with respect to LASIK, as presented in Fig. 3.6. Central nerve fibers are detectable at 1 week and after SMILE (Fig. 3.6), and a rapid gain of central nerve fiber density can be observed by IVCM.

Another reason for less nerve fiber damage in SMILE in comparison to LASIK may correlate to the higher level of collateral damage and decellularization of keratocytes induced by the excimer laser [34, 36]. It is not clear yet whether viable keratocytes are needed to sustain corneal nerve function or vice versa, but prolonged keratocyte apoptosis and acellularity have been observed after excimer laser-based techniques in which an extended period of postoperative denervation is common [34, 37]. As mentioned earlier, some stromal nerve fibers directly innervate stromal keratocytes [13]. Both structures probably mediate the complex wound healing pattern occurring after keratorefractive laser procedures and are likely to be involved in the delicate system aimed to restore the corneal integrity, transparency, and epithelial dynamics after surgery.

3.4   Keratocyte Changes After ReLEx® Refractive Surgery: In Vivo Evaluation and Wound Healing Patterns

The immediate postoperative stromal modification of LASIK or surface ablation is dominated by the laser-tissue interaction and the keratocyte-mediated wound healing cascade. These events are known to actively influence the refractive outcome and optical transparency of the cornea particularly in surface ablation procedures. There is a specific type of inflammation and wound healing [38] with a central role of keratocyte apoptosis in activation of the wound healing cascade effecting corneal nerves, lacrimal glands, and tear film [7].

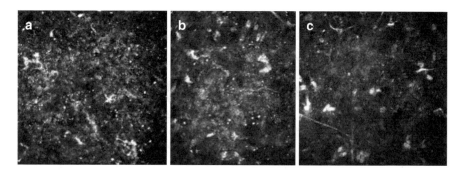

Fig. 3.7 IVCM images of SMILE lamellar interface at different intervals after surgery. (**a**) Stroma interface 1 week after SMILE shows increased matrix reflectivity, apoptotic keratocytes, bright reflective particles, and mild edema. (**b**) One month after surgery, viable keratocyte nuclei are visible along with improved reflectivity. (**c**) At 6 months after surgery, the interface appears stable, with rare keratocytes interspersed and linear structure of a regenerating nerve fiber. Keratocyte density is always reduced at the interface

Keratocyte activation stimulated by LASIK has a short duration compared with that reported after surface ablation techniques. Regardless of the method used for flap creation, the stromal tissue presents early morphological changes in keratocytes located below the flap, at the edge of the photoablation [38] (see also Fig. 3.2). However, the presence of this new virtual space—"the surgical interface"—allows the collection of liquid or particles as well as the spread of inflammatory cells.

IVCM morphology of the stromal interface (either in LASIK and SMILE) is characterized by the discontinuity of the stromal cellular architecture. Examples of microscopic characteristics of ReLEx® stromal interfaces are shown in (Fig. 3.7).

The interface is generally imaged microscopically as a poorly cellulated layer within the anterior stroma, with variable amount of reflective debris and particles clearly distinguishable from the other corneal layers [39]. A typical feature at the interface, which has been confirmed by IVCM, is the lower cellular activity and stromal remodeling. It has been shown that "acellular zones" are present on both sides of the interface [40] and appear thicker when investigated in the first days after surgery, whereas keratocytes are visible closer to the interface in the following weeks [41]. The keratocyte-free layers probably represent zone undergoing apoptosis or necrosis, an assumption supported by histological investigation [42].

IVCM analysis of SMILE interface and stromal keratocyte changes over time are presented in (Fig. 3.8).

In ReLEx® surgery keratocyte apoptosis is mostly confined in the stromal sublayer adjacent to the extracted lenticules, and surrounding tissue is generally affected by minimal apoptotic/necrotic effect and inflammation, in the early postoperative period. If surgical excessive manipulation and irrigation of the interface are performed during surgery, a certain degree of stromal edema, with packed keratocytes within fluid cystic spaces, can be observed by IVCM in the first days after procedure. These features may not be clearly evident at slit lamp examination and can be responsible for delayed visual recovery, often observed in the first week (Fig. 3.9a). The interface and the

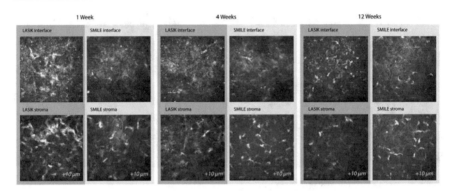

Fig. 3.8 IVCM images showing the interface and stromal keratocyte characteristics after SMILE and Fs-LASIK. In the *first row*, confocal images of the lamellar interface comparing LASIK and SMILE at different time course are presented. SMILE interfaces generally show lower degree of bright particles and present visible keratocyte nuclei, indicating lower apoptosis. The *second row* presents images of the stromal layers immediately below the interface (+10 μm), showing greater keratocytes activation in the first weeks after surgery (probably related to the excimer ablation effects in addition to the femtosecond laser dissection). Keratocytes distribution tends to equal after 3 months after surgery

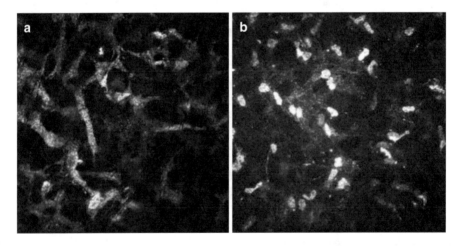

Fig. 3.9 (**a**) Stromal postoperative edema with cystic extracellular spaces (honeycomb pattern) and packed keratocytes with increased reflectivity. (**b**) Activated keratocytes in the anterior stroma characterized by bright nuclei and visible cytoplasmic processes

adjacent layers generally become transparent few days after surgery, and keratocyte response generally persists mild to moderate, as compared with excimer laser ablations (Fig. 3.8). Fs-LASIK also exerts an excimer ablation effect in addition to the femtosecond laser dissection compared with SMILE, and this is probably related to the greater keratocytes activation observed for few weeks after surgery (Fig. 3.8). Keratocyte stability probably equals that of SMILE at 3 months (Mastropasqua L,

Nubile M. 2015). The occurrence of persistent keratocytes activation, which may be responsible for abnormal collagen deposition and optical degradation of the interface quality in SMILE, is a rare phenomenon and generally can be reversed by prolonged use of steroid eye drops similar to excimer laser surgery (Fig. 3.9b).

3.5   Summary

In vivo findings suggest that surgical denervation is significantly less in SMILE as compared to other laser refractive procedures. Also a faster nerve regeneration is likely to occur after SMILE. These advantages are thought to be related to the neuroanatomy of the cornea and to the particular flap-less procedure of the SMILE technique. However, also in SMILE nerve fibers intersecting the lenticule-cap plane become transected by the femtosecond laser cut and degenerate thereafter, reducing the overall central corneal nerve fibers density. This damage appears significantly less as compared to flap-based and surface ablation techniques, in which the fiber resection is almost total.

After SMILE, some of the spared stromal fibers run over the lenticule plane, in the mid-periphery, piercing the BL outside the treatment area and therefore remain intact and contributing to the subbasal central plexus. Based on these observations, SMILE surgery favors a better preservation of the corneal neural architecture and a greater postoperative corneal sensitivity leading to a lower incidence and course of the neurotrophic epitheliopathy.

Keratocytes apoptosis, stromal inflammation, and secondary keratocyte activation are seen as mild to moderate, without substantial differences in any intrastromal refractive techniques. Thus, an abnormal healing compromising the optical quality of the lamellar interface and of the remaining stroma is unlikely to occur.

References

1. Sutton GL, Kim P (2010) Laser in situ keratomileusis in 2010 – a review. Clin Experiment Ophthalmol 38(2):192–210
2. Reynolds A, Moore JE, Naroo SA, Moore CB, Shah S (2010) Excimer laser surface ablation – a review. Clin Experiment Ophthalmol 38(2):168–182
3. Ang EK, Couper T, Dirani M, Vajpayee RB, Baird PN (2009) Outcomes of laser refractive surgery for myopia. J Cataract Refract Surg 35(5):921–933
4. Arba-Mosquera S, Klinner T (2014) Improving the ablation efficiency of excimer laser systems with higher repetition rates through enhanced debris removal and optimized spot pattern. J Cataract Refract Surg 40(3):477–484
5. Sakimoto T, Rosenblatt MI, Azar DT (2006) Laser eye surgery for refractive errors. Lancet 367(9520):1432–1447
6. O'Brart DP (2014) Excimer laser surface ablation: a review of recent literature. Clin Exp Optom 97(1):12–17
7. Dupps WJ Jr, Wilson SE (2006) Biomechanics and wound healing in the cornea. Exp Eye Res 83(4):709–720
8. Rózsa AJ, Beuerman RW (1982) Density and organization of free nerve endings in the corneal epithelium of the rabbit. Pain 14(2):105–120

9. Müller LJ, Marfurt CF, Kruse F, Tervo TM (2003) Corneal nerves: structure, contents and function. Exp Eye Res 76(5):521–542
10. Al-Aqaba MA, Fares U, Suleman H, Lowe J, Dua HS (2010) Architecture and distribution of human corneal nerves. Br J Ophthalmol 94(6):784–789
11. Shaheen BS, Bakir M, Jain S (2014) Corneal nerves in health and disease. Surv Ophthalmol 59(3):263–285
12. He J, Bazan NG, Bazan HE (2010) Mapping the entire human corneal nerve architecture. Exp Eye Res 91(4):513–523
13. Müller LJ, Pels L, Vrensen GF (1996) Ultrastructural organization of human corneal nerves. Invest Ophthalmol Vis Sci 37(4):476–488
14. Wilson SE, Chaurasia SS, Medeiros FW (2007) Apoptosis in the initiation, modulation and termination of the corneal wound healing response. Exp Eye Res 85(3):305–311
15. West-Mays JA, Dwivedi DJ (2006) The keratocyte: corneal stromal cell with variable repair phenotypes. Int J Biochem Cell Biol 38(10):1625–1631
16. Chiou AG, Kaufman SC, Kaufman HE et al (2006) Clinical corneal confocal microscopy. Surv Ophthalmol 51:482–500
17. Dhaliwal JS, Kaufman SC, Chiou AG (2007) Current applications of clinical confocal microscopy. Curr Opin Ophthalmol 18:300–307
18. Villani E, Baudouin C, Efron N et al (2014) In vivo confocal microscopy of the ocular surface: from bench to bedside. Curr Eye Res 39(3):213–231
19. Nubile M, Mastropasqua L (2009) In vivo confocal microscopy of the ocular surface: where are we now? Br J Ophthalmol 93(7):850–852
20. Meng ID, Kurose M (2013) The role of corneal afferent neurons in regulating tears under normal and dry eye conditions. Exp Eye Res 117:79–87
21. Hovanesian JA, Shah SS, Maloney RK (2001) Symptoms of dry eye and recurrent erosion syndrome after refractive surgery. J Cataract Refract Surg 27(4):577–584
22. Ambrósio R Jr, Tervo T, Wilson SE (2008) LASIK-associated dry eye and neurotrophic epitheliopathy: pathophysiology and strategies for prevention and treatment. J Refract Surg 24(4):396–407
23. Zhang F, Deng S, Guo N, Wang M, Sun X (2012) Confocal comparison of corneal nerve regeneration and keratocyte reaction between FS-LASIK, OUP-SBK, and conventional LASIK. Invest Ophthalmol Vis Sci 53(9):5536–5544
24. Erie JC, McLaren JW, Hodge DO, Bourne WM (2005) Recovery of corneal subbasal nerve density after PRK and LASIK. Am J Ophthalmol 140(6):1059–1064
25. Pérez-Santonja JJ, Sakla HF, Cardona C, Chipont E, Alió JL (1999) Corneal sensitivity after photorefractive keratectomy and laser in situ keratomileusis for low myopia. Am J Ophthalmol 127(5):497–504
26. Murphy PJ, Corbett MC, O'Brart DP, Verma S, Patel S, Marshall J (1999) Loss and recovery of corneal sensitivity following photorefractive keratectomy for myopia. J Refract Surg 15(1):38–45
27. De Paiva CS, Chen Z, Koch DD, Hamill MB, Manuel FK, Hassan SS, Wilhelmus KR, Pflugfelder SC (2006) The incidence and risk factors for developing dry eye after myopic LASIK. Am J Ophthalmol 141(3):438–445
28. Albietz JM, Lenton LM, McLennan SG (2004) Chronic dry eye and regression after laser in situ keratomileusis for myopia. J Cataract Refract Surg 30(3):675–684
29. Albietz JM, Lenton LM (2004) Management of the ocular surface and tear film before, during, and after laser in situ keratomileusis. J Refract Surg 20(1):62–71
30. Patel SV, McLaren JW, Kittleson KM, Bourne WM (2010) Subbasal nerve density and corneal sensitivity after laser in situ keratomileusis: femtosecond laser vs mechanical microkeratome. Arch Ophthalmol 128(11):1413–1419
31. Wei S, Wang Y (2013) Comparison of corneal sensitivity between Fs-LASIK and femtosecond lenticule extraction (ReLEx FLEx) or small-incision lenticule extraction (ReLEx SMILE) for myopic eyes. Graefes Arch Clin Exp Ophthalmol 251(6):1645–1654

32. Vestergaard AH, Grønbech KT, Grauslund J, Ivarsen AR, Hjortdal JØ (2013) Subbasal nerve morphology, corneal sensation, and tear film evaluation after refractive femtosecond laser lenticule extraction. Graefes Arch Clin Exp Ophthalmol 251(11):2591–2600

33. Li M, Niu L, Qin B, Zhou Z, Ni K, Le Q, Xiang J, Wei A, Ma W, Zhou X (2013) Confocal comparison of corneal reinnervation after small incision lenticule extraction (SMILE) and femtosecond laser in situ keratomileusis (Fs-LASIK). PLoS One 8(12):e81435

34. Mohamed-Noriega K, Riau AK, Lwin NC, Chaurasia SS, Tan DT, Mehta JS (2014) Early corneal nerve damage and recovery following small incision lenticule extraction (SMILE) and laser in situ keratomileusis (LASIK). Invest Ophthalmol Vis Sci 55(3):1823–1834

35. Reinstein DZ, Archer TJ, Randleman JB (2013) Mathematical model to compare the relative tensile strength of the cornea after PRK, LASIK, and small incision lenticule extraction. J Refract Surg 29:454–460

36. Riau AK, Angunawela RI, Chaurasia SS, Lee WS, Tan DT, Mehta JS (2011) Early corneal wound healing and inflammatory responses after refractive lenticule extraction (ReLEx). Invest Ophthalmol Vis Sci 52:6213–6221

37. Erie JC, Patel SV, McLaren JW, Hodge DO, Bourne WM (2006) Corneal keratocyte deficits after photorefractive keratectomy and laser in situ keratomileusis. Am J Ophthalmol 141:799–809

38. Alio JL, Javaloy J (2013) Corneal inflammation following corneal photoablative refractive surgery with excimer laser. Surv Ophthalmol 58(1):11–25

39. Vesaluoma M, Pérez-Santonja J, Petroll WM et al (2000) Corneal stromal changes induced by myopic LASIK. Invest Ophthalmol Vis Sci 41:369–376

40. Erie JC, Nau CB, McLaren JW et al (2004) Long-term keratocyte deficits in the corneal stroma after LASIK. Ophthalmology 111:1356–1361

41. Vesaluoma MH, Petroll WM, Perez-Santonja JJ et al (2000) Laser in situ keratomileusis flap margin: wound healing and complications imaged by in vivo confocal microscopy. Am J Ophthalmol 130:564–573

42. Dong Z, Zhou X, Wu J, Zhang Z, Li T, Zhou Z, Zhang S, Li G (2014) Small incision lenticule extraction (SMILE) and femtosecond laser LASIK: comparison of corneal wound healing and inflammation. Br J Ophthalmol 98(2):263–269

Part II

Clinical Development and Current Techniques

Brief Historical Overview of the Clinical Development of ReLEx® Surgical Procedure

4

Marcus Blum and Walter Sekundo

Content

Corneal resectional refractive procedures for the correction of myopia were pioneered by Barraquer and Ruiz [1]. They removed a layer of intrastromal tissue utilizing a microkeratome and called this procedure "in situ keratomileusis." However, the results of the procedure performed with mechanical devices were not entirely satisfactory [2, 3].

Few years later, lasers entered the field of refractive surgery, and in 1989, Stern reported the use of lasers to ablate the cornea [4]. The first use of a laser instead of a microkeratome to achieve an intrastromal lenticule was described in 1996 [5]. Using a picosecond laser, an intrastromal lenticule was generated and was then removed manually after lifting the flap. In two highly myopic eyes, a fair amount of manual dissection was required resulting in an irregular surface [6]. Its use was therefore limited to animal studies [7, 8]. It is noteworthy that in the early 1990s of the last century, the idea of full femtosecond laser system-based refractive correction had already been born.

M. Blum, MD (✉)
Department of Ophthalmology, Helios Hospital Erfurt, Erfurt, Germany
e-mail: marcus.blum@helios-kliniken.de

W. Sekundo, MD
Department of Ophthalmology, Philipps University of Marburg and Universitätsklinikum Giessen & Marburg GmbH, Marburg, Germany

© Springer International Publishing Switzerland 2015
W. Sekundo (ed.), *Small Incision Lenticule Extraction (SMILE):*
Principles, Techniques, Complication Management, and Future Concepts,
DOI 10.1007/978-3-319-18530-9_4

47

Fig. 4.1 The treatment pack

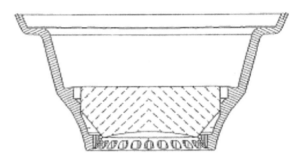

First clinical results with a laser-induced extraction of a refractive lenticule were reported with five blind or amblyopic eyes in 2003 [9]. Unfortunately, these first studies lack a sufficient number of eyes and a detailed analysis of the achieved refractive data. The studies have not been continued with a representative study cohort.

For several years, the advanced femtolaser systems were restricted to the creation of flaps as a replacement for mechanical microkeratomes, while the actual refractive procedure remained the domain of the 193 nm-ArF-excimer laser [10]. With regard to the quality of the surgical outcome, femtosecond laser microkeratomes have advantages over mechanical devices [11–13].

After several years of an intensive laboratory research, a prototype femtosecond laser system – now known as VisuMax® – was developed by Carl Zeiss Meditec AG, Jena, Germany. In order to enable intraoperative target fixation by the patient, an illuminated and curved treatment interface (so-called contact glass) that does not elevate the intraocular pressure above the diastolic blood pressure was developed and tested beforehand on animals (Fig. 4.1) and in human volunteers (obviously without treatment). Mainly because the suction is applied at the cornea rather than at the sclera (as with other fs-lasers), the IOP raises to only 70–80 mmHg [14, 15]. This enables patients to see the blinking target and results in a good centration preventing clinically relevant induction of high-order aberrations (HOA) [16]. Furthermore, the "gentle corneal interface" concept with its low suction and a continuous fixation target may reduce potential risks for the posterior segment [17]. To prove the function of the VisuMax fs-laser as a femto microkeratome, a study combining the fs-flap cut with the MEL 80 excimer laser ablation was performed parallel to the further development of FLEx procedure described below [18].

During this period of time in 2005, a series of studies by Blum and Sekundo (unpublished data) on animals, blind and amblyopic eyes, underwent a new refractive procedure, which no longer required an excimer laser (Fig. 4.2). The procedure was called femtosecond lenticule extraction (FLEx) in order to distinguish it from other known refractive procedures. In autumn of 2006, during the American Academy of Ophthalmology Meeting in Las Vegas/USA, Sekundo and Blum

Fig. 4.2 A photograph from the first animal experiments testing femtosecond lenticule extraction

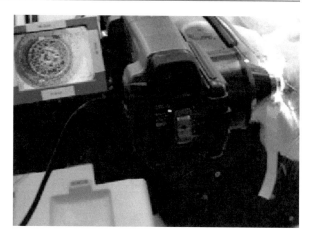

presented the very first ten cases of corneal refractive correction using a prototype of the VisuMax® femtosecond laser. The first peer-reviewed article was published by Sekundo et al. in 2008 [19]. Animation images of the procedure reproduced from the first award-winning surgical video shown by Sekundo and Blum at the 2008 ASCRS Meeting in Chicago are summarized in Fig. 4.3.

A cohort of fully seeing eyes treated for myopia and myopic astigmatism followed this very first report. A total of 108 eyes had been recruited and treated from 56 patients with spherical myopia between −2 and −8.5 D and myopic astigmatism up to −6 D cyl. These eyes were followed up for 6 months and – on a voluntary basis – for 12 months [20, 21]. Meanwhile, 5-year results of this initial cohort have been published [22].

In this first larger series, the intended flap thickness varied between 110 and 160 μm; the flap diameter was chosen between 7.0 and 8.5 mm. In all 108 cases, a superior hinge, 50° in chord length, was left. The lenticule diameter varied between 6.0 and 7.3 mm according to patient's scotopic pupil diameter. No nomograms were available at the beginning, and a special equation (Patent No. DE 102006053120 A1) based on Mannerlyn's formula was used to calculate the geometry and the thickness of the refractive lenticule. The postoperative regimen consisted of preservative-free antibiotic, steroid, and hyaluronic acid lubricating drops four times per day each for 1 week. Keeping in mind that this first prospective clinical study started without a nomogram, the results of 98.1 % of eyes within 1 D of refractive target were satisfactory and exceeded our expectations.

Shah was the third surgeon in the world who took up the ReLEx technique and significantly contributed to its development in the early phase of this procedure. Her main achievement was not only to optimize laser settings for the 200 kHz machine used at this stage of development in a substantial number of patients but also to realize that also the laser scan (or cut) direction matters [23].

Following the successful implementation of FLEx, the next aim was to further develop a surgical procedure in which a flap no longer was necessary. This procedure was named small incision lenticule extraction (SMILE): by passing a dissector through a small 2–3 mm incision, the anterior and posterior lenticular interfaces are separated, and the lenticule is then removed through the incision (Fig. 4.4). This eliminates the need to create a flap, and the cornea above the upper interface of the lenticule is now referred to as the cap. The first surgical video of SMILE was shown during the Cataratta refractiva in Milano in 2009. However, it took another 3 years till peer-reviewed publications appeared in the scientific literature [24, 25]. The first larger series of eyes operated with the SMILE technique was published by Sekundo and Blum et al. and, unlike in today's SMILE, was carried out through two opposite

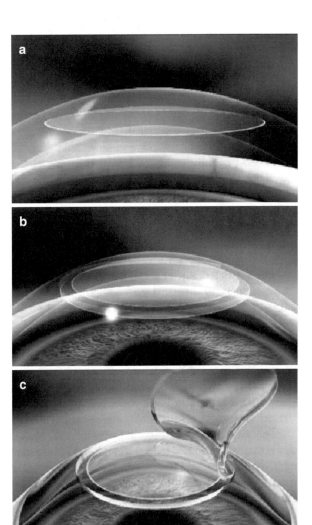

Fig. 4.3 A schematic drawing of the FLEx procedure. The VisuMax® femtosecond laser system cuts the back of the refractive lenticule (**a**) followed by its front surface incision (**b**) followed by a vertical incision leaving an arc of 50° untouched (hinge). The final step is performed manually, with the flap beeing lifted (**c**) with the spatula and the lenticule removed manually using forceps (**d**). The flap is then repositioned (**e**)

Fig. 4.3 (continued)

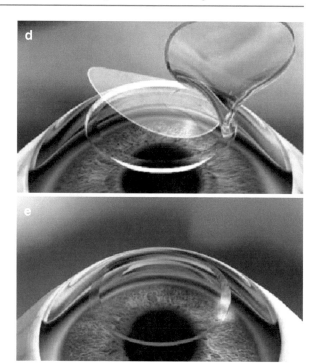

entering incisions, 4 mm each [24]. A total of 91 eyes clearly demonstrated the "prove of principle," and the encouraging results motivated a number of researchers to test the new surgical technique [25–27]. This resulted in a variety of smaller changes in surgical technique, but the main elements remained unchanged: the laser first created the lower interface, followed by the upper interface of the lenticule either using an out-to-in direction or using an in-to-out direction. Shah was the first surgeon to use a single-entering incision [25], and it was also her who systematically worked toward very small incision used today.

Although the refractive results were good in the first study (very close to those observed in LASIK), visual recovery time was slightly longer. The effect of different scanning patters, optimization of energy parameters, and spot-spacing settings led to much improved visual recovery times [23, 26, 28, 29]. Furthermore, a 500-kHz-laser was released and the precision of lenticule creation was improved [30, 31]. In terms of safety and complications, SMILE has also been shown to be quite outstanding [32]. Meanwhile, first results are also available for the treatment of hyperopia (see Chap. 19). After 2010–2011, the technique became increasingly popular, and many outstanding surgeons joined the "SMILE community" improving the quality of this procedure step by step. It is a pleasure to have many of these surgeons as coauthors of this book sharing their view of the present and the future of "all-in-one" femtosecond laser surgery.

Fig. 4.4 A schematic drawing oft he SMILE procedure. The VisuMax femtosecond laser system cuts the lenticule (**a**) followed by a small incision (**b**). The lenticule is removed through the small insision (**c**)

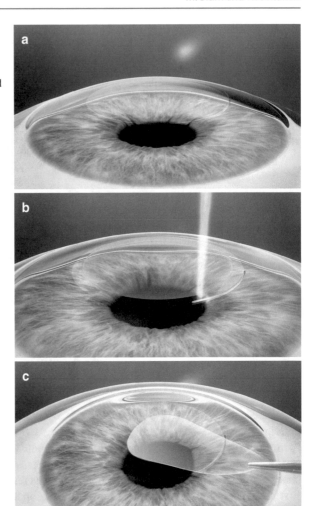

References

1. Barraquer JI (1996) The history and evolution of keratomileusis. Int Ophthalmol Clin 36:1–7
2. Ibrahim O, Waring GO, Salah T, el Maghraby A (1995) Automated in situ Keratomileusis for myopia. J Refract Surg 11:431–441
3. Wiegand W, Krusenberg B, Kroll P (1995) Keratomileusis in situ bei hochgradiger Myopie. Erste Ergebnisse. Ophthalmologe 92:402–409
4. Stern D, Schoenlein RW, Puliafito CA (1989) Corneal ablation by nanosecond, picoseconds, and femtosecond lasers at 532 and 625 nm. Arch Ophthalmol 107:567–592
5. Ito M, Quantock AJ, Malhan S, Schanzlin DJ, Krueger RR (1996) Picosecond laser in situ keratomileusis with a 1053-nm Nd:YFL laser. J Refract Surg 12:721–728
6. Krueger RR, Juhasz T, Gualano A, Marchi V (1998) The picosecond laser for nonmechanical laser in situ keratomileusis. J Refract Surg 14:467–469

7. Kurtz RM, Horvath C, Liu HH, Krueger RR, Juhasz T (1998) Lamellar refractive surgery with scanned intrastromal picoseconds and femtosecond laser pulses in animal eyes. J Refract Surg 14:541–548

8. Heisterkamp A, Mamon T, Kermani O, Drommer W, Welling H, Ertmer W, Lubatschowski H (2003) Intrastromal refractive surgery with ultrashort laser pulses: in vivo study on the rabbit eye. Graefes Arch Clin Exp Ophthalmol 241:511–517

9. Ratkay-Traub I, Ferincz IE, Juhasz T, Kurtz RM, Krueger RR (2003) First clinical results with the femtosecond neodymium-glass laser in refractive surgery. J Refract Surg 19:94–103

10. Nordan LT, Slade SG, Baker RN (2003) Femtosecond laser flap creation for laser in situ keratomileusis: six-months follow-up of the initial US clinical series. J Refract Surg 19:8–14

11. Kezirian GM, Stonecipher KG (2004) Comparison of the IntraLase femtosecond laser and mechanical microkeratome for laser in situ keratomileusis. J Cataract Refract Surg 30:26–32

12. Durrie DS, Kezirian GM (2005) Femtosecond laser versus mechanical keratome flaps in wavefront-guided laser in situ keratomileusis: prospective contralateral eye study. J Cataract Refract Surg 31:120–126

13. Tran DB, Sarayba MA, Bor Z et al (2005) Randomized prospective clinical study comparing induced aberrations with IntraLase and Hansatome flap creation in fellow eyes: potential impact on wavefront-guided laser in situ keratomileusis. J Cataract Refract Surg 31:97–105

14. Vetter JM, Holzer MP, Teping C, Weingartner WE, Gericke A, Stoffelns B, Pfeiffer N, Sekundo W (2011) Intraocular pressure during corneal flap preparation: comparison among four femtosecond lasers in porcine eyes. J Refract Surg 27:427–433

15. Vetter JM, Faust M, Gericke A, Pfeiffer N, Weingärtner WE, SEkundo W (2012) Intraocular pressure measurements during flap preparation using 2 femtosecond lasers and 1 microkeratome in human donor eyes. J Cataract Refract Surg 38:2011–2018

16. Sekundo W, Gertnere J, Bertelmann T, Solomatin I (2014) One-year refractive results, contrast sensitivity, high-order aberrations and complications after myopic small-incision lenticule extraction (ReLEx SMILE). Graefes Arch Clin Exp Ophthalmol 252(5):837–843

17. Reviglio VE, Kuo IC, Gramajo L et al (2007) Acute rhegmatogenous retinal detachment immediately following laser in situ keratomileusis. J Cataract Refract Surg 33:536–539

18. Blum M, Kunert K, Gille A, Sekundo W (2009) First experience in femtosecond LASIK with the Zeiss VISUMAX® laser. J Refract Surg 25:350–356

19. Sekundo W, Kunert K, Russmann C, Gille A, Bissmann W, Strobrawa G, Stickler M, Bischoff M, Blum M (2008) First efficacy and safety study of femtosecond lenticule extraction for the correction of myopia. J Cataract Refract Surg 34:1513–1520

20. Blum M, Kunert K, Schröder M, Sekundo W (2010) Femtosecond lenticule extraction (FLEX) for the correction of myopia: 6 months results. Graefes Arch Clin Exp Ophthalmol 248: 1019–1027

21. Blum M, Kunert KS, Engelbrecht C, Dawczynski J, Sekundo W (2010) Femtosekunden-Lentikel-Extraktion (FLEX) – Ergebnisse nach 12 Monaten bei myopem Astigmatismus. Klin Monatsbl Augenheilkd 227:961–965

22. Blum M, Flach A, Kunert KS, Sekundo W (2014) Five-year results of refractive lenticule extraction. J Cataract Refract Surg 40:1425–1429

23. Shah R, Shah S (2011) Effect of scanning patterns on the results of femtosecond laser lenticule extraction refractive surgery. J Cataract Refract Surg 37:1636–1647

24. Sekundo W, Kunert K, Blum M (2011) Small incision femtosecond lenticule extraction (SMILE) for the correction of myopia and myopic astigmatism: results of a 6 months prospective study. Br J Ophthalmol 95:335–339

25. Shah R, Shah S, Segupta S (2011) Results of small incision lenticule extraction: all-in-one femtosecond laser refractive surgery. J Cataract Refract Surg 37:127–137

26. Hjortdal JO, Vestergaard AH, Ivarsen A, Ragunathan S, Asp S (2012) Predictors for the outcome of small-incision lenticule extraction for Myopia. J Refract Surg 28:865–871

27. Kamiya K, Shimizu K, Igarashi A, Kobashi H (2014) Visual and refractive outcomes of femtosecond lenticule extraction and small-incision lenticule extraction for myopia. Am J Ophthalmol 157:128–134

28. Kunert KS, Blum M, Duncker GIW, Sietmann R, Heichel J (2011) Surface quality of human corneal lenticules after femtosecond laser surgery for myopia comparing different laser parameters. Graefes Arch Clin Exp Ophthalmol 249:1417–1424
29. Heichelt J, Blum M, Duncker GIW, Sietmann R, Kunert KS (2011) Surface quality of porcine corneal lenticules after Femtosecond Lenticule Extraction. Ophthalmic Res 46:107–112
30. Reinstein DZ, Archer TJ, Gobbe M (2013) Accuracy and reproducibility of cap thickness in small incision lenticule extraction. J Refract Surg 29:810–815
31. Ozgurhan EB, Agca A, Bozkurt E, Gencer B, Celik U, Cankaya KI, DEmirok A, Yilmaz OF (2013) Accuracy and precision of cap thickness in small incision lenticule extraction. Clin Ophthalmol 7:923–926
32. Ivarsen A, Asp S, Hjortdal J (2014) Safety and complications of more than 1500 small incision lenticule extraction procedures. Ophthalmology 121:822–882

Current Technique and Instrumentation for SMILE

5

Ekktet Chansue

Contents

The ReLEx® SMILE procedure is typically performed under topical anesthesia and can be divided into two steps: the femtosecond laser application and the manual removal of the lenticule. The femtosecond laser cuts are intrastromal, without any external corneal wound, and subsequently can be performed in a "clean" fashion, i.e., no disinfection needed. The second step requires sterility of the field.

> **Bilateral Surgery**
> The procedure can be performed bilaterally provided that the patient has been properly counseled and has gone through proper informed consent process. For bilateral ReLEx SMILE, the procedure can be performed either as two sequential unilateral procedures (complete laser cuts and lenticule extraction

No financial interest in any device or instrument mentioned in this chapter.

Electronic supplementary material The online version of this chapter (doi:10.1007/978-3-319-18530-9_5) contains supplementary material, which is available to authorized users.

E. Chansue, MD
TRSC International LASIK Center, Bangkok, Thailand
e-mail: echansue@gmail.com

© Springer International Publishing Switzerland 2015
W. Sekundo (ed.), *Small Incision Lenticule Extraction (SMILE):
Principles, Techniques, Complication Management, and Future Concepts*,
DOI 10.1007/978-3-319-18530-9_5

in one eye, then the same in the other) or as a step-wise bilateral operation (sequential laser cuts in both eyes, followed by sequential lenticule extraction in both eyes).

The advantages of completing the whole procedure one eye at a time are:

- More conventional feel
- Simpler setup of the operating room. Less manpower needed

The advantages of doing each step bilaterally are:

- This clearly separates the "clean" and the "sterile" parts of the procedure, making contaminations less likely.
- The extraction of the lenticules can be performed with another microscope, freeing the laser bed for the preparation of the next patient. This is especially useful in high-flow practices, with adequate manpower in the operating room.
- The laser treatments occur in rapid succession, decreasing the risks of overdehydration of the surface of the second eye, which may lead to slow visual recovery and possibly variations in refractive results.
- Uneventful completion of femtosecond laser cuts in both eyes helps ensure that lenticule extraction can be successfully performed in both eyes. Should there be any problem in the laser part of the procedure in either eye, the surgeon and the patient have the option of proceeding or aborting the procedure.

5.1   Femtosecond Laser Application

Much like the setting of the excimer laser in LASIK, the surgeon is ultimately responsible in setting up parameters of the laser to get optimum results. The details of the femtosecond laser settings are discussed elsewhere in this textbook (see Chaps. 1 and 11).

The procedure involving the docking and the application of the laser cuts are similar to that in FemtoLASIK flap creation. The difference is that FemtoLASIK flap cuts only involve two cuts (the planar cut and the edge cut), whereas ReLEx® SMILE involves four cuts: (a) the posterior plane cut, (b) the lenticule edge cut, (c) the anterior plane cut, and (d) the entrance wound cut (Fig. 5.1). Consequently it takes roughly twice the duration (about 30 s) to complete the ReLEx cuts, compared to flap cuts.

This is the most critical part of the procedure refractively because it is where the femtosecond laser defines the anterior and posterior plane between which the lenticule will be created. The dimension and shape of the lenticule determine the amount

Fig. 5.1 Femtosecond laser ReLEx(R) cuts, (**a**) frontal, and (**b**) cross-section views

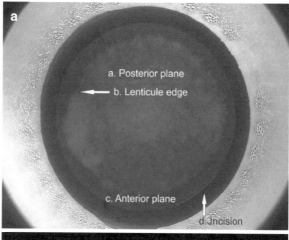

a. Posterior plane

b. Lenticule edge

c. Anterior plane

d. Incision

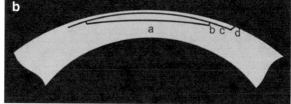

Fig. 5.2 The second eye is taped shut before the laser application to the first eye

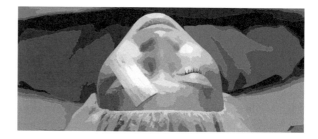

of spherical and cylindrical correction and the effective optical zone of treatment. The smoothness of the cuts affects the smoothness of the corneal surface once the lenticule has been extracted. The smoothness of the surface is further affected by the postoperative epithelial remodeling (see Chap. 13), but the initial smoothness immediately after the procedure has significant effects on the early visual quality and recovery.

In bilateral cases, while the first eye is receiving the laser treatment, the second eye should be held shut with an adhesive strip, to prevent uneven dehydration of the epithelium that may lead to temporary roughness of the surface, in turn affecting the smoothness of the laser cuts and the visual recovery time (Fig. 5.2).

5.2   Lenticule Extraction

Immediately after the femtosecond laser cuts are completed, the lenticule is still not freely extractable, as there are still micro-bridges between the interfaces. The surgeon breaks those micro-bridges by bluntly dissecting in the plane between the lenticule and the stromal cap and that between the lenticule and the stromal bed, to free the lenticule from its surroundings. The lenticule is then retrieved and removed from the pocket.

Instrumentation

The Lenticule Extraction part of ReLEx® SMILE requires minimal instrumentation. This includes:

Basic instruments: Eyelid speculum, absorbent surgical spears, sterile balanced salt solution (15 cc bottle), blunt irrigating cannula, and Kelman-McPherson-type forceps.

An eyelid speculum: A solid-bladed, self-retaining speculum. I prefer the pediatric size, as the shorter blades create more vertical space resulting in a roughly hexagonal, rather than rectangular, exposure. This is especially useful in the eyes with shorter palpebral fissures (Fig. 5.6). In the eyes with better exposed globes, a standard LASIK aspirating speculum in the aspirating mode (connected to the pump) during the laser cut will help to prevent tear pooling and reduce the incidence of suction loss. Wire speculum should be avoided.

Specific instruments: Lenticule dissector for freeing the lenticule and microforceps for retrieving the freed lenticule.

Meanwhile some further modification of different instruments were made by other surgeons in cooperation with other ophthalmic instruments manufacturers, but they are generally speaking either:

The Chansue ReLEx® Dissector

When I started performing ReLEx® in 2010, the standard instrument recommended by the laser manufacturer for dissecting the lenticule was the Seibel flap lifter (Fig. 5.3) or a simple phako spatula and the Blum modified McPherson forceps. As the name implies, Seibel flap lifter was designed to be used for flap lifting in FemtoLASIK. It worked quite well as a dissector for ReLEx® FLEX, as the flap and the lenticule were lifted in the same manner as the flap in FemtoLASIK. However, the instrument lends itself poorly to lenticule dissection when a small incision is intended, as it is too straight and too long. Consequently, I designed a new instrument specifically for ReLEx®

lenticule dissection later that year. It has a curved tapering circular shaft which ends in a conical semi-blunt dissecting tip. The other end of the dissector bears a Sinskey-style hook in the same fashion as does the Seibel Flap Lifter but is slightly longer to facilitate the delineation of both planes. The instrument is called the Chansue ReLEx® Dissector (CRD). The CRD was designed to conform with average corneal curvature, to minimize distortion and stress to the anterior stromal cap (Fig. 5.4a).

Fig. 5.3 The Seibel LASIK flap lifter

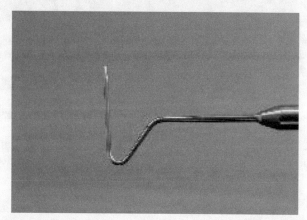

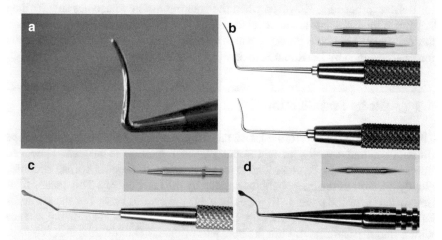

Fig. 5.4 (**a**) The Chansue ReLEx(R) Dissector (CRD). (**b**) Kostin spatulas (Medin-Ural/Russia) are slightly slender compared to the original Chansue dissector and is produced in two different lengths. (**c**) The original Blum spoon (Geuder GmbH/Germany) designed at the early stage of ReLEx® development features a semi-sharp ending similar to a hockey knife. (**d**) Due to a better laser cut quality of the 500 kHZ VisuMax®, Bloom spoon was replaced by several similar instruments featuring a blunt, rounded, and polished head as shown in this advanced Chansue dissector

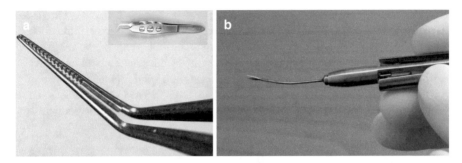

Fig. 5.5 (**a**) McPherson serrated forceps (Geuder GmbH, Germany) modified by Blum is a simple forceps for lenticule extraction for entering incisions of 2.5 mm or longer. (**b**) The Advanced Lenticule Forceps

1. Spatulas resembling the CRD, but with different lengths and diameter (e.g., Kostin spatula/Medin-Ural/Russia, Fig. 5.4b) or
2. Dissectors featuring a combination of the CRD and Blum spoon (e.g., Tan dissector/ASICO/USA, Güell dissector/Geuder Germany, Reinstein single-use dissector/Malosa/UK). See also Fig. 5.4c, d.

Lenticule-retrieving microforceps. Marcus Blum's modified McPherson forceps with serrated jaws (Fig. 5.5a) was the first lenticule retrieving instrument designed for ReLEx® procedure. However, when the entering incision becomes smaller than 2.5 mm, a microforceps is recommended. The standard microforceps instrument is the Advanced Lenticule Forceps, which is a modification of the Shah Lenticule forceps, designed by Dr. Rupal Shah in 2011 (Fig. 5.5b).

5.3   Globe Stabilization

The dissection can be performed with the patient self-fixating on the microscope illuminator, and usually no additional physical fixation is needed. However, immediately after the femtosecond laser application, the central cornea becomes cloudy because of the microbubbles created by the laser energy. This makes fixation difficult for the patient. To partially clear the central cornea of these microbubbles, pointed pressure can be applied on the central corneal epithelial surface with a smooth instrument. I use the heel part of the CRD to do this, as it provides a small pressure point and the smoothness of its surface prevents epithelial disturbances. This allows the microscope light to get through the cornea and helps the patient fixate (Fig. 5.7). Some surgeons feel more comfortable to manually stabilize the globe with the nondominant hand using either a micro-spear sponge or Thorton's fixating ring for contra-pressure or a colibri style forceps to hold the globe (see Fig. 5.15).

5.4   Dissecting Efficiency

The dissector has the highest dissecting power at the tip. The quality of the femto-second laser cuts in the previous step determines how effectively the dissector separates the interfaces. In some eyes, the dissector can only advance a few millimeters with each sweep of the dissecting tip, whereas in others, just one sweep will separate the whole expanse of the pocket.

5.5   Surgical Steps

1. Sterile field with routine disinfection and draping of the upper half of the face. Some surgeons also prefer to drape the eyelids and the eyelashes.
2. Placement of eyelid speculum (Fig. 5.6).
3. Pointed pressure in the center of the cornea, just enough to create a relatively clear stroma through which the patient can see the microscope light and fixate. The patient is instructed to fixate on the light at all times (Fig. 5.7).
4. The hook end of the CRD is used to break the entrance wound open (Fig. 5.8).
5. A small pocket (1×2 mm) is made with the hook. While doing the planar dissection of this pocket, care should be taken to keep the most distal part of the hook parallel to the corneal surface (or pointed slightly up and away from the eye) to ensure that this pocket is located anterior to the lenticule (Fig. 5.9).
6. The CRD is then rotated so that the tip of the hook is pointed down toward the center of the eyeball. The tip is then pressed down and pushed across centripetally in a tangential direction. This action helps the tip find the edge of the lenticule. Only 1 mm-long separation is sufficient to serve as a marker for the

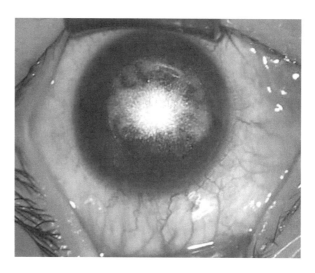

Fig. 5.6 The short blades of the pediatric eyelid speculum create hexagonal exposure

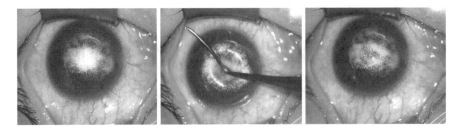

Fig. 5.7 Central microbubbles are pushed away by pointed pressure on the epithelial surface, creating a relatively clear area though which the patient can fixate at the microscope illuminator

Fig. 5.8 Creating the incision

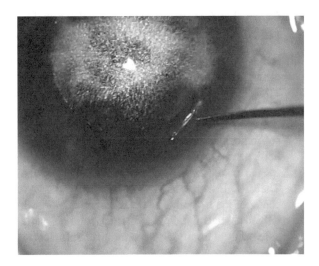

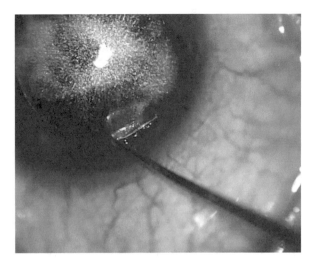

Fig. 5.9 A small pocket is created with the hook. The tip of the hook is pointed upward in an attempt to stay in the plane anterior to the lenticule

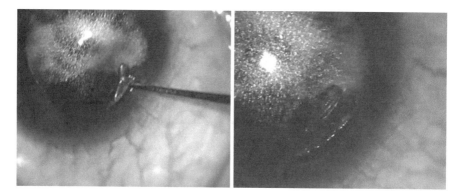

Fig. 5.10 *Left*: Locating the edge of the lenticule ensures that the two planes are positively identified. *Right*: Partially separated edge of the lenticule is visible under the cap

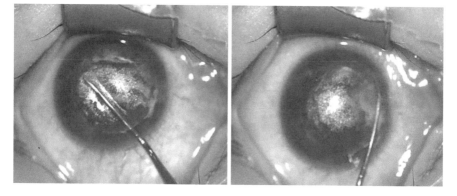

Fig. 5.11 Sweeping motion of the dissector is created by the rotation of the handle. The surgeon moves his/her hand position back and forth to maintain pivot at the small incision

lenticule edge. This step ensures that the instrument is in the correct plane before the dissection of the anterior (cap-lenticule) interface is started (Fig. 5.10).

7. Once the lenticule edge has been located, the dissecting end of the CRD is used to separate the anterior plane (Fig. 5.11).
8. Going under the lenticule edge identified in step 6, the CRD is then used to dissect the posterior plane to free the lenticule from its stromal bed (Fig. 5.12).
9. The patient is then instructed to look down and the lenticule forceps are used to remove the freed lenticule from the stromal pocket (Fig. 5.13).
10. Optionally the pocket may be irrigated to wash out debris or foreign bodies such as epithelial cells. This also floats up the cap and lets it oppose evenly back to the stromal bed, minimizing irregularity in the cap (Fig. 5.14).

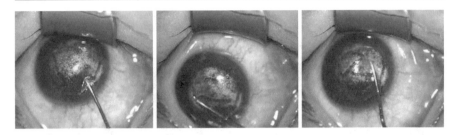

Fig. 5.12 Posterior plane dissection to free the lenticule

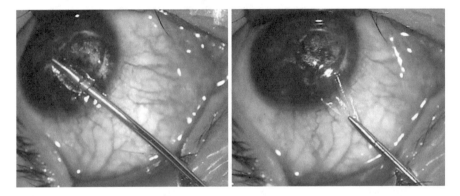

Fig. 5.13 The lenticule is removed from the pocket with a pair of microforceps

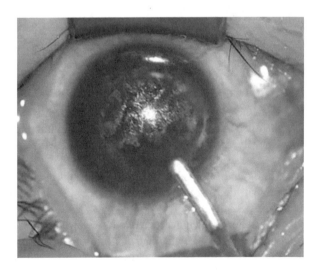

Fig. 5.14 Irrigating the pocket

5.6   Variations in Instrumentation and Technique

Manual globe fixation. In patients who are not able to self-fixate on the microscope light, manual globe fixation can be useful. This can be in the form of a single-point fixation with a pair of toothed forceps (Fig. 5.15), or with a ring-type fixator such as the Fine-Thornton ring.

ReLEx® SMILE is still a relatively new procedure. As more surgeons perform this procedure, there are bound to be variations both in the instrumentation and the surgical technique. The following are only a few examples of the presently performed variations.

Double entrance. Some surgeons advocate the use of two entrance incision cuts about 90° apart. An extra entrance can act as a "safety net" in case of problems at the other entrance. It can also act as an exit incision to push the freed lenticule through and obviate the need of lenticule forceps.

Liquid infiltration method. Some surgeons find that using balanced salt solution to wet the interface makes for easier dissection.

There are also other methods and dissector designs being used effectively by various surgeons around the world, and the reader is referred to the surgical video library enclosed with this book.

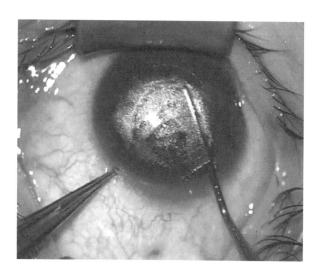

Fig. 5.15 Manual globe fixation with 0.12 toothed forceps

Refining Results with SMILE: Tips and Tricks

6

Sri Ganesh

Contents

Surgery is both a science and an art, which should blend seamlessly with technology in today's world. This is particularly so with refractive surgery and ReLEx® SMILE. Lenticule extraction with VisuMax femtosecond laser technology (Carl Zeiss Meditec, Jena, Germany) is a relatively new procedure, which is emerging as the preferred practice for correcting myopia and myopic astigmatism due to its various advantages over the current available techniques.

Any new technique has a learning curve and understanding small nuances will help improve outcomes. It is observed that results with SMILE vary from center to

Financial Disclosure The author is a consultant for Carl Zeiss Meditec AG and receives study and travel support from Carl Zeiss Meditec AG.

Electronic supplementary material The online version of this chapter (doi:10.1007/978-3-319-18530-9_6) contains supplementary material, which is available to authorized users.

S. Ganesh, MS, DNB
Department of Phaco Refractive, Nethradhama Super Speciality Eye Hospital,
Bangalore, India
e-mail: phacomaverick@gmail.com

center and surgeon to surgeon especially the first postoperative day outcomes. The visual recovery is influenced by ease of dissection and time taken for surgery. In my experience of over 2,500 surgeries in the past 2 years, I have made some observations which have helped refine my technique and improve patient outcomes. I have set about trying to elaborate some of these tips in this chapter which would help the beginner in SMILE surgery gain mastery over the procedure.

6.1   The Environment

The laser room environment is critical for excimer laser surgery and both temperature and humidity should be maintained at optimal levels. The VisuMax femtosecond laser is more robust and less sensitive to changes in humidity and temperature [1], but I have found that maintaining a temperature of around 22 °C and humidity of 50 % is optimal and gives the best tissue dissection. A lower temperature affects the fluence and the bubble pattern, which may make dissection of the tissue planes more difficult.

6.2   Optimal Fluence (Laser Energy)

The laser energy is of utmost importance to get a good bubble pattern and greatly influences the ease of dissection and surgical time [2]. The spot size and spacing is fixed and the newer software has a spot spacing of 4.5 μ, which has improved the dissection of the deeper plane. The general tendency is to increase the laser energy when dissection is difficult, but this may be counterproductive with the VisuMax femtosecond laser and give rise to more opaque bubble layer (OBL).

It is important to carefully observe the OBL pattern and make necessary changes in the fluence levels to get an optimal bubble layer. If you notice a fast OBL – the OBL occurs preceding or during the spiral pattern of the laser wave – the energy is high and needs to be reduced (Fig. 6.1). A slow OBL, which occurs after the laser dissection, is seen if the fluence is lower and indicates that the energy may have to be increased (Fig 6.2). A perfect bubble layer is observed at optimal laser energy with no OBL and a uniform density of the bubble layer (Fig 6.3). Generally this is obtained for most VisuMax® lasers between fluence levels of 32 and 35 (160–175 nanojoules). The VisuMax® is programmed to perform the deeper plane dissection from periphery to center (spiral in) first, followed by the side cut and then the superficial plane dissection from center to periphery (spiral out), and lastly the access incision. This provides for minimum tissue distortion and longer period of patient fixation. The high frequency of the VisuMax (500 kHz) performs good tissue dissection at lower energy with less tissue distortion (for further information on energy management, see Chap. 11).

Fig. 6.1 Fast OBL (opaque bubble layer)

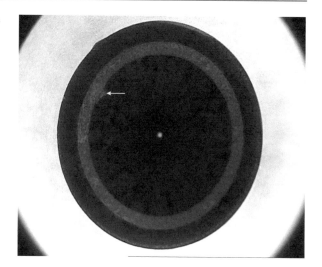

Fig. 6.2 Slow OBL

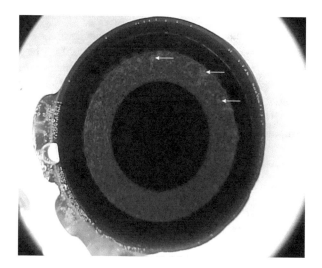

6.3   Patient Positioning

The VisuMax® laser has a curved interface which applanates the patient's cornea with a low corneal suction. The advantage of this system is that patient fixation is maintained even after suction is applied and incidence of subconjunctival hemorrhage is negligible, but the downside is higher incidence of suction loss. Any obstruction to the movement of the gantry will result in a higher incidence of suction loss during the procedure, and this can be avoided by proper patient positioning before applanation and suction application.

Fig. 6.3 Normal bubble
pattern

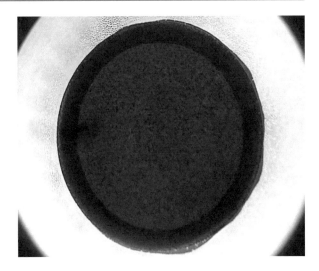

Proper exposure can be attained by elevating the chin and turning the face in the opposite direction. The head rest of the VisuMax® bed can be moved up and down to obtain an optimal chin elevation, without making the patient uncomfortable.

This maneuver is particularly useful in patients having a prominent nose, and it is prudent to ensure that there is a clear gap from the patient's nose and laser gantry before corneal applanation and suction. It is also important to orient the suction tube temporally.

6.4 Nomogram Adjustment

Results vary with every laser and every surgeon, and it is imperative that all surgeons develop a nomogram adjustment to refine their results. I have found that there is a tendency for undercorrection with my initial results of SMILE. The refraction is also pupil dependent [3], and I like to add 10 % to myopic astigmatic treatments in patients who are between 20 and 30 years and if scotopic pupil size is larger than 6 mm.

6.5 Astigmatism Correction

The VisuMax® does not have cyclotorsion compensation, but it is important to correct for cyclotorsion in higher cylinders. Cyclotorsion can occur for various reasons [4]: (1) cyclotorsion occurring naturally from sitting to supine position, (2) positioning of head and turning the face, (3) speculum and patient's resistance to it and Bell's phenomenon, and (4) applanation and suction can induce cyclotorsion due to difference in the corneal curvature and curvature of the interface.

Manual compensation for cyclotorsion: The 0–180° axis is marked on the limbus extending about 2 mm on either side onto the cornea with the patient sitting upright. Take care so that the marking does not extend into the optical zone of the laser as this may interfere with the laser delivery and make dissection tougher. Following applanation and suction, check for the alignment of the 0–180 marks with respect to the horizontal line on the reticule of the microscope ocular or the VisuMax screen, then rotate the patient interface (suction cup) so that it is aligned before proceeding with the laser delivery (Video 6.1).

I prefer to correct for cyclotorsion in cases where the cylindrical power is greater than 0.5 D. I also like to overcorrect astigmatism by 10 % as per my nomogram correction and use an optical zone of more than 6.5 mm. This gives me a good postoperative outcome even in high cylinders and pure astigmatism.

6.6 Applanation and Suction

Angle kappa and centration: VisuMax does not have pupil centration and tracking. The centration is along the patient's line of sight and may be away from the pupil center if the patient has a large angle kappa. Asking the patient to look at the microscope light gives an idea about the angle kappa apart from the preoperative topography, which will also give this information. This is important in patients who have a large angle kappa as after applanation and suction you may find the centration away from the pupil center and you may unnecessarily try to undock and correct for this. Patient fixation and centration along the line of sight gives a better centration of the corneal flattening and visual outcomes than pupil centration [5].

After draping and inserting the speculum, observe for pooling of fluid (tears, BSS, anesthetic) in the fornices. Remove the excess fluid with a sponge; otherwise, this may predispose to suction loss. Avoid drying the cornea excessively as this can again hamper applanation and docking. It is important not to touch the applanating surface of the patient interface as any stains can reduce laser delivery and cause black areas in the bubble pattern which can make dissection difficult.

Applanate the cornea slowly and steadily while asking the patient to fixate on the green flashing fixation light. After applanating the cornea about 80 %, apply suction to get a good dock. It is very important to converse with the patient and tell them what to expect. Explain that the green fixation will disappear once the deeper pass of the laser happens and they should hold their gaze steady without searching for the green light. Also give a countdown of the time. This vastly reduces the incidence of suction loss and improves patient experience. Most cases of suction loss occur after the deep laser pass when fixation disappears and patients try searching for the green light. The surrounding area of the suction cup should be dry. If you notice any leak of fluid, which is characterized by a darkening of the white surrounding area and escape of bubbles (Fig. 6.4), it is better not to proceed with the laser treatment. Release the vacuum, dry the fornices and conjunctiva and the suction cup, or replace the suction cup and re-dock to get a good vacuum seal before proceeding with the laser treatment.

Fig. 6.4 Leaking fluid and bubbles during suction loss

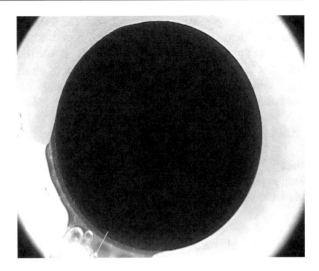

Some patients have loose bulbar conjunctiva, which can prolapse toward the cornea and increase the incidence of suction loss. This also can block the laser delivery especially the incision at 12 o'clock position. In such cases, it is better to use a solid blade speculum and applanate the cornea fully before putting on the suction.

6.7   Dissection of the Lenticule

Adjust magnification and illumination to clearly visualize the incision. Using a fixation forceps stabilizes the globe and prevents sudden movements. It also provides for countertraction during dissection, making it easier and faster. I like to use a corneal fixation forceps which offers a two-point fixation in my left hand and a ReLEx pocketing hook/separator in my right hand (Fig. 6.5). Once the incision is opened up, the gas bubbles clear up to quite an extent and the patient is able to fixate on the microscope light. Identification of the superficial and deep planes is very important.

I like to initially identify and separate the superficial plane on the left side of the incision and the deeper plane on the right side of the incision so that entry into the planes is specific. I dissect the superficial plane first and then the deeper plane. While dissecting the deeper plane, I like to leave a little tissue bridge undissected on one side (usually the right) and then dissect the other side completely. This offers countertraction and prevents the lenticule from rolling over. The dissector is moved in a winshield wiper – like fashion with the fulcrum at the incision. This prevents extension and tear of the incision especially in small incisions (2 mm). The lenticule is grabbed with a micro forceps near the edge of the tissue bridge and separated in a rhexis-like motion.

Once the lenticule is removed, place it on the cornea and spread it out and inspect it to see if it is complete and edges are intact and circular. This is especially

Fig. 6.5 Fixation forceps
and tissue dissection

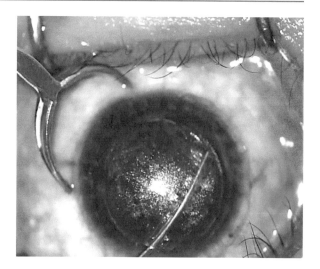

indicated if there is OBL and difficult dissection. The slit lamp on the VisuMax® can be used to inspect the cornea and side cut to look for any remnants of the lenticule.

I prefer to irrigate the interface gently and minimally with BSS as I find that this improves visual recovery and results in better first-day vision. I dry the incision with a Merocel® sponge before removing the speculum.

In my experience, the bubble pattern, ease of dissection, and time taken for dissection influence the first-day postoperative visual recovery.

Having a systematic approach, individual nomograms, and ensuring an easy and fast dissection with minimal tissue handling will ensure good visual outcomes, and ReLEx SMILE may offer a paradigm shift in the way refractive surgery is performed, having all the advantages of LASIK and safety of PRK with the greatest patient comfort.

References

1. Lubatschowski H (2008) Overview of commercially available femtosecond lasers in refractive surgery. J Refract Surg 24(1):S102–S107
2. Dupps WJ Jr, Wilson SE (2006) Biomechanics and wound healing in the cornea. Exp Eye Res 83:709–720
3. Iseli HP, Bueeler M, Hafezi F, Seiler T, Mrochen M (2005) Dependence of wavefront refraction on pupil size due to the presence of higher order aberrations. Eur J Ophthalmol 15:680–687
4. Chang J (2008) Cyclotorsion during laser in situ keratomileusis. J Cataract Refract Surg 34:1720–1726
5. Pande M, Hillman JS (1993) Optical zone centration in keratorefractive surgery: entrance pupil centre, visual axis, coaxially sighted corneal reflex, or geometric corneal centre? Ophthalmology 100:1230–1237

Overview of Clinical Results for Low and Moderate Myopia

7

Kimiya Shimizu, Kazutaka Kamiya, Akihito Igarashi, Hidenaga Kobashi, Rie Ikeuchi, and Walter Sekundo

Contents

7.1   Introduction

During the last few years, small-incision lenticule extraction (SMILE) has become clinically available in Europe and Asia as an alternative to LASIK for correction of myopia. In the United States, the procedure is currently undergoing clinical trials for approval by the US Food and Drug Administration. In SMILE, a femtosecond laser is used to create an intrastromal lenticule that is manually extracted through a small peripheral incision (see Chap. 5) [1, 2]. Being flap-free, this surgical approach may

K. Shimizu, MD, PhD (✉) • K. Kamiya • A. Igarashi • H. Kobashi • R. Ikeuchi
Department of Ophthalmology, University of Kitasato School of Medicine,
1-15-1 Kitasato, Minami, Sagamihara, Kanagawa 252-0374, Japan
e-mail: kimiyas@med.kitasato-u.ac.jp

W. Sekundo
Department of Ophthalmology, Philipps University of Marburg and Universitätsklinikum
Giessen & Marburg GmbH, Marburg, Germany

© Springer International Publishing Switzerland 2015
W. Sekundo (ed.), *Small Incision Lenticule Extraction (SMILE):
Principles, Techniques, Complication Management, and Future Concepts*,
DOI 10.1007/978-3-319-18530-9_7

Fig. 7.1 Appearance of a LASIK-treated eye 10 years post-op. Superficial punctate keratitis is clearly visible after fluorescein staining

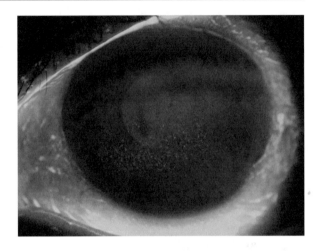

After SMILE   After LASIK

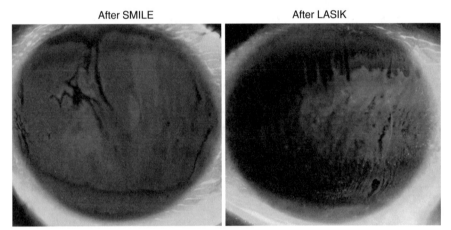

Fig. 7.2 Eyes underwent small-incision lenticule extraction (SMILE) and LASIK 1 year post-op. The SMILE procedure has a less pronounced impact on the ocular surface compared with LASIK

reduce some of the side effects of LASIK, such as dry eye (Fig. 7.1), flap dislocation [3], reduced sensitivity and subbasal nerve fiber density (see Chap. 3) [4], and corneal ectasia [5]. The efficacy, predictability, and safety of the procedure have been reported to be on par with femtosecond LASIK [1, 2, 6–9]. However, some studies report a relatively high percentage of eyes with loss of two or more lines in visual acuity [6], and only a few studies have reported complications related to SMILE surgery [10, 11]. Furthermore, SMILE has some advantages over LASIK in dry eye parameters and subjective symptoms, postoperatively (Fig. 7.2) [12, 13]. This review evaluates the early clinical outcomes after SMILE technique in patients with low to moderate myopia; however the vast majority of published results are focused on moderate myopia [1, 2, 14–21]. Only one study on low myopia by Reinstein et al. was found in peer-reviewed literature [21]. It will be discussed separately. In addition, presented but not yet published 5-year results will be shared with the reader.

7.2   Trial Evaluation

Data source articles limited to SMILE were searched in the following databases from January 2011 to December 2014: PubMed (Medline). A minimum follow-up of 3 months was required. Eyes with the mean preoperative spherical equivalent (SE) of more than −6.0 diopters (D) were excluded from this review. The data of interest for each clinical outcome were extracted as follows: (1) *Efficacy*: the number of eyes achieving an uncorrected distance visual acuity (UDVA) of 20/20 or better postoperatively. (2) *Predictability*: the number of eyes achieving a postoperative spherical equivalent (SE) within ±0.50 diopter (D) of the intended target. (3) *Safety*: the number of eyes that lost two or more lines of postoperative CDVA relative to the preoperative CDVA. (4) *Stability*: the changes in manifest refraction from 1 week to the last follow-up.

7.3   Recent Findings

Eleven studies, mostly on SMILE for moderate myopic correction and one study on low myopia were included in this review and summarized in Table 7.1.

Table 7.1 Summary of clinical results after small-incision refractive lenticule extraction in eyes with low to moderate myopia

Study[a] (year)	No. of eyes	Follow-up (month)	Mean Preop SE (D)	UDVA ≥20/20 (%)	Eyes within ±0.5 D (%)	Lost ≥2 lines in CDVA (%)	Change in SE (D)
Sekundo [1] (2011)	91	6	−4.75±1.56	83.5	80.2	2.2	0.05
Shah [2] (2011)	51	6	−4.87±2.16	62	91	0	−0.06±0.27
Kamiya [14] (2014)	26	6	−4.21±1.63	96	100	0	0.00±0.30
Ganesh [15] (2014)	50	3	−4.37±2.21	96	NA	0	NA
Ang [16] (2014)	20	3	−3.23±1.09	65.0	65.0	NA	NA
Lin [17] (2014)	60	3	−5.13±1.75	85.0	98.3	1.7	NA
Xu [18] (2015)	52	12	−5.53±1.70	83	90.4	0	−0.06±0.37
Sekundo [19] (2014)	54	12	−4.68±1.29	88	92	0	−0.19±0.19
Agca [20] (2014)	40	12	−4.03±1.61	65	95	0	−0.33±0.25
Kunert [21] (2015)	55	12	−4.66±1.75			1.8	−0.11±0.42
Reinstein [22] (2014)	110	12	**−2.61±0.55**	96	84	0	−0.05±0.36

SE spherical equivalent, *D* diopters, *UDVA* uncorrected distance visual acuity, *CDVA* corrected distance visual acuity, *NA* data not available

[a]First author

7.3.1 Efficacy

Efficacy data was reported by all 11 studies that qualified for inclusion in this review. The percentage of eyes with an UDVA of 20/20 or better at the last follow-up visit was 62–92 % in previous studies.

7.3.2 Predictability

Predictability data was reported by 10 of the 11 studies that qualified for inclusion in this review. The percentage of eyes with an SE of ±0.50 D at the last follow-up visit was 65–100 % in previous studies.

7.3.3 Safety

Safety data was reported by 10 of the 11 studies that qualified for inclusion in this review. The percentage of eyes with lost two or more lines in CDVA was 0–2.2 % in previous studies.

7.3.4 Stability

Stability data was reported by 8 of the 11 studies that qualified for inclusion in this review. The mean change in manifest refraction from 1 week to the last follow-up was −0.06 to 0.05 D in previous studies.

7.3.4.1 Low Myopia

So far only one single study was published on true low myopia. This very recent study by Reinstein et al. [22] looked at 110 eyes with a preoperative spherical equivalent of −2.61 ± 0.54 D and a range of −1.03 to −3.5 D. Two surgeons using fairly large optical zones with an average of 7.01 mm treated a rather young population with a mean age of 32.4 years (Table 7.1).

7.4 Discussion

At the beginning of the learning curve, treatment of higher myopias is recommended, as the extraction of a thick lenticule is manually less demanding and the results of high myopias treated with SMILE supersede the results obtained by FS-LASIK at this refractive error (see Chap. 9). Thus, many clinicians, particularly those not personally familiar with SMILE technology, believe SMILE to be a technique for high refractive errors only. Our brief review supports the continued use of SMILE for treatment of low to moderate myopia. Overall, refractive and visual outcomes of the SMILE procedure are as good for the correction of low to moderate myopia as

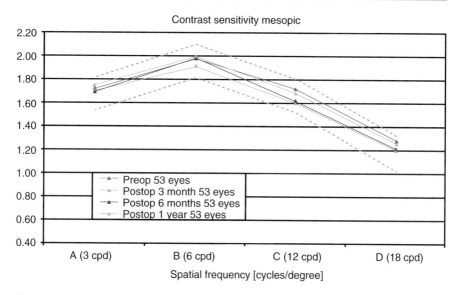

Fig. 7.3 An example of mesopic contrast sensitivity after SMILE for moderate myopia showing virtually no difference to pre-op values at 1 year follow-up (From Sekundo et al. [19])

excimer-based treatments. The reader should study Table 7.1, carefully keeping in mind that the first two studies by Sekundo et al. and Shah et al. were performed with the old 200 kHz laser. It is also true for the latter study of Kunert et al. [21] as it gives a 12-month follow-up partially on the same cohort of patients as initially reported by Sekundo et al. [19]. It is striking that the results obtained for lower degree of myopia with the current 500 kHz laser are definitely not inferior to those obtained with excimer laser. The SMILE procedure has a potential to supersede excimer surface ablation as the treatment of choice even for the correction of low to moderate myopia in patients with a high risk of eye trauma or those who simply do not want to have a flap, as today's patients are quite aware of biomechanical risks associated with flap creation. In addition, more postoperative comfort and no fear to touch the eye anytime after surgery are appealing arguments. Contrast sensitivity values are at least as good as after excimer-based surgery and sometimes are even better, in particular when looking at high-order aberration (Fig. 7.3). In this regard, the Reinstein et al. [22] study is of particular interest, because the authors treated true low myopias of −3.5 D or less. The little helpful "tricks" for safe low myopic SMILE surgery are (a) to increase the optical zone, (b) to increase the minimum lenticule thickness from the preset 15 μm to 20 or 25 μm, and (c) to increase the transition zone. The knowledge of a better biomechanical tensile strength after SMILE easily justifies these measures of thickening the lenticule (see Chap. 13). The first 5-year results of the initial cohort treated by Blum and Sekundo in 2009 (and published in 2011) were presented by K. Täubig at the meeting of the German Ophthalmological Society (DOG) in September of 2014. All of the 60 eyes with mid myopia treated 5 years ago had a remarkable refractive stability (Fig. 7.4), provided the patients were >25 years old.

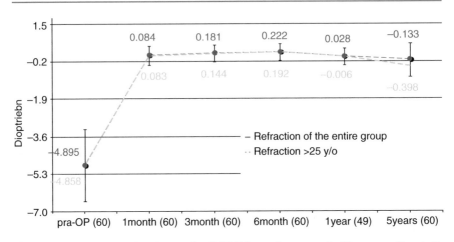

Fig. 7.4 Stability of refraction 5 years after SMILE for moderate myopia. Please note: Four individuals younger than 25 years are fully responsible for the regression of the entire group (−0.25 D) implicating a known fact of increasing axial myopia at this age (Courtesy of Prof. Blum)

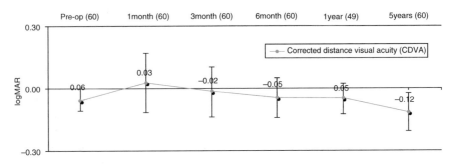

Fig. 7.5 The best corrected distance visual acuity displays a further improvement over the course of 5 years (Courtesy of Prof. Blum)

Further improvement of UDVA and CDVA beyond the preoperative level was noticed (Fig. 7.5). So what is the lowest level of myopia that can be safely treated by current 500 kHz technology? We believe that this question should be asked differently: How thick shall we make our lenticule in order to safely extract it? Reinstein et al. went as thin as 51 μm and there were some oral presentation claiming that 40 μm can also be safely extracted, when the energy settings are adapted (Dr B. Meyer, personal communication). In our subjective opinion, 50 μm as a "rule of thumb" should be enough for a very experienced SMILE. Novel surgeons should not take any additional risks with the current 500 kHz VisuMax® technology.

References

1. Sekundo W, Kunert KS, Blum M (2011) Small incision corneal refractive surgery using the small incision lenticule extraction (SMILE) procedure for the correction of myopia and myopic astigmatism: results of a 6-month prospective study. Br J Ophthalmol 95:335–339
2. Shah R, Shah S, Sengupta S (2011) Results of small incision lenticule extraction: all-in-one femtosecond laser refractive surgery. J Cataract Refract Surg 37:127–137
3. Iskander NG, Peters NT, Anderson Penno E, Gimbel HV (2001) Late traumatic flap dislocation after laser in situ keratomileusis. J Cataract Refract Surg 27:1111–1114
4. Pérez-Santonja JJ, Sakla HF, Cardona C et al (1999) Corneal sensitivity after photorefractive keratectomy and laser in situ keratomileusis for low myopia. Am J Ophthalmol 127:497–504
5. Geggel HS, Talley AR (1999) Delayed onset keratectasia following laser in situ keratomileusis. J Cataract Refract Surg 25:582–586
6. Hjortdal JØ, Vestergaard AH, Ivarsen A et al (2012) Predictors for the outcome of small-incision lenticule extraction for myopia. J Refract Surg 28:865–871
7. Vestergaard A, Ivarsen AR, Asp S, Hjortdal JØ (2012) Small-incision lenticule extraction for moderate to high myopia: predictability, safety, and patient satisfaction. J Cataract Refract Surg 38:2003–2010
8. Vestergaard A, Ivarsen A, Asp S, Hjortdal JØ (2013) Femtosecond (FS) laser vision correction procedure for moderate to high myopia: a prospective study of ReLEx flex and comparison with a retrospective study of FS-laser in situ keratomileusis. Acta Ophthalmol 91:355–362
9. Kamiya K, Igarashi A, Ishii R, Sato N, Nishimoto H, Shimizu K (2012) Early clinical outcomes, including efficacy and endothelial cell loss of refractive lenticule extraction using a 500 kHz femtosecond laser to correct myopia. J Cataract Refract Surg 38:1996–2002
10. Dong Z, Zhou X (2013) Irregular astigmatism after femtosecond laser refractive lenticule extraction. J Cataract Refract Surg 39:952–954
11. Sharma R, Vaddavalli PK (2013) Implications and management of suction loss during refractive lenticule extraction (ReLEx). J Refract Surg 29:502–503
12. Li M, Zhao J, Shen Y, Li T, He L, Xu H, Yu Y, Zhou X (2013) Comparison of dry eye and corneal sensitivity between small incision lenticule extraction and femtosecond LASIK for myopia. PLoS One 8, e77797
13. Gao S, Li S, Liu L, Wang Y, Ding H, Li L, Zhong X (2014) Early changes in ocular surface and tear inflammatory mediators after small-incision lenticule extraction and femtosecond laser-assisted laser in situ keratomileusis. PLoS One 9, e107370
14. Kamiya K, Shimizu K, Igarashi A, Kobashi H (2014) Visual and refractive outcomes of femtosecond lenticule extraction and small-incision lenticule extraction for myopia. Am J Ophthalmol 157:128–134
15. Ganesh S, Gupta R (2014) Comparison of visual and refractive outcomes following femtosecond laser- assisted lasik with smile in patients with myopia or myopic astigmatism. J Refract Surg 30:590–596
16. Ang M, Mehta JS, Chan C, Htoon HM, Koh JC, Tan DT (2014) Refractive lenticule extraction: transition and comparison of 3 surgical techniques. J Cataract Refract Surg 40:1415–1424
17. Lin F, Xu Y, Yang Y (2014) Comparison of the visual results after SMILE and femtosecond laser-assisted LASIK for myopia. J Refract Surg 30:248–254
18. Xu Y, Yang Y (2015) Small-incision lenticule extraction for myopia: results of a 12-month prospective study. Optom Vis Sci 92(1):123–131
19. Sekundo W, Gertnere J, Bertelmann T, Solomatin I (2014) One-year refractive results, contrast sensitivity, high-order aberrations and complications after myopic small-incision lenticule extraction (ReLEx SMILE). Graefes Arch Clin Exp Ophthalmol 252(5):837–843

20. Ağca A, Demirok A, Cankaya Kİ, Yaşa D, Demircan A, Yildirim Y, Ozkaya A, Yilmaz OF (2014) Comparison of visual acuity and higher-order aberrations after femtosecond lenticule extraction and small-incision lenticule extraction. Cont Lens Anterior Eye 37:292–296
21. Kunert KS, Melle J, Sekundo W, Dawczynski J, Blum M (2015) Ein-Jahres-Ergebnisse bei Small-Incision-Lentikel-Extraktion (SMILE) zur Myopiekorrektur. (One-year results of small incision lenticule extraction (SMILE) in myopia). Klin Monbl Augenheilkd 232(1):67–71
22. Reinstein DZ, Carp GI, Archer TJ, Gobbe M (2014) Outcomes of small incision lenticule extraction (SMILE) in low myopia. J Refract Surg 30:812–818

Astigmatism Correction

8

Marcus Blum and Walter Sekundo

Content

The dome shape of the cornea is spherical as long as all the meridians have the same curvature. In astigmatism the refractive power of the cornea varies in its vertical and horizontal meridians, and therefore a point image of a point object cannot be formed. The meridians of maximum and minimum curvature are called the principal meridians, and in regular astigmatism these are at 90° to each other. From the curvature of the cornea, the mean corneal power and the cylinder power can be calculated, and clinically this is described by the axis of the cylinder and its power in dioptres (D) [1].

Depending on the orientation of the principal meridians, different types of astigmatism can be distinguished:

- *With-the-rule astigmatism*: the vertical meridian has higher refractive power (90° ± 15°).
- *Against-the-rule astigmatism* (so called because it occurs less frequently): the horizontal meridian has higher refractive power (0° ± 15° or 180° ± 15°).
- *Oblique astigmatism:* the principal meridians are tilted by an angle between 15° and 75° (or 105° and 165°) but are still perpendicular to each other.

M. Blum, MD (✉)
Department of Ophthalmology, Helios Hospital Erfurt, Erfurt, Germany
e-mail: marcus.blum@helios-kliniken.de

W. Sekundo, MD
Department of Ophthalmology, Philipps University of Marburg and Universitätsklinikum Giessen & Marburg GmbH, Marburg, Germany

© Springer International Publishing Switzerland 2015
W. Sekundo (ed.), *Small Incision Lenticule Extraction (SMILE):*
Principles, Techniques, Complication Management, and Future Concepts,
DOI 10.1007/978-3-319-18530-9_8

It is clear that refractive error is not static through life. The highest incidence of astigmatism (up to 65 %) is reported in the first year of life [2]. The decrease in astigmatism demonstrated over the first years in life appears to be a result of the increase in eye size and flattening of the cornea [3]. By adulthood, this high incidence of astigmatism has disappeared. The incidence of astigmatism greater than 1.0 D in adults is reported in up to 8 % of patients [4].

Several surgical concepts have been tested for the therapy of astigmatism. Astigmatic keratotomy (AK) and limbal relaxing incisions (LRIs) became popular as these procedures can be used in combination with cataract surgery [5]. Recent generations of excimer lasers provide an effective surgical technique to correct astigmatism with satisfactory results. However, the excimer laser treatment of spherical myopia has been shown to be more predictable than the correction of myopic astigmatism [6].

One study reported surgically induced astigmatism by corneal flap making. Huang et al. found an average of 0.12 D with-the-rule astigmatism induced after LASIK with a superior hinge [7]. The conclusion was that the astigmatic shift is an effect of the circular keratotomy and the absence of the keratotomy at the site of the superior hinge. The superior hinge causes a steepening of the astigmatism on the 90° axis, while the circular keratotomy causes a reduction of corneal astigmatism overall. However, there is a lack of vector-based studies in the literature, and other authors could not find this evidence.

Within a short period of time, continuous improvements of the ReLEx technique led to comparable results with regard to safety and stability of the refractive results [8–12].

However, the current "benchmark" for astigmatism correction is modern excimer lasers, some of them with a dynamic cyclotorsional eye tracker. In contrast, femtosecond lasers work on an eye fixed by a suction "contact glass". Thus, the accuracy of applying suction without globe rotation is of an upmost importance to a proper axial alignment during the treatment. Kunert and co-authors gave the first detailed report on astigmatism treatment using vector analysis [13]. A vector analysis was done on the refractive data, which mainly followed the definitions and formulas given by Eydelman and co-workers [14].

Her study evaluated the efficacy, predictability and safety of the all-femto-procedure ReLEx® FLEx for correction of myopic astigmatism. A complete set of refractive data of 182 treatments (87 left and 95 right eyes) for the follow-up periods of 1 week and 1, 3 and 6 months is reported. The study consisted of 182 eyes of 113 patients with spherical myopia between 0 D and −8.75 D (MV −4.10 D, SD=1.51 D) and myopic astigmatism between −0.25 D and −6.0 D (MV 0.96 D, SD±0.87 D). The data set encompassed treatments of sphere and astigmatism. Vector analysis was performed to study the astigmatic results at each follow-up visit. The data allow a quantitative analysis of under- and overcorrection. The slope of the linear regression lines expresses the factor of over- and undercorrection. All over the four follow-up periods of 1 week and 1, 3 and 6 months, the factors amount to 0.96, 0.89, 0.91 and 0.88, respectively. This data corresponds to undercorrections of 4 %, 11 %, 9 % and 12 %, respectively, as shown in the table below.

		C ≤ 0.25 D	0.25 D $<C$ ≤ 0.5 D	0.5 D $<C$ ≤ 0.75 D	0.75 D $<C$ ≤ 1 D	1 D $<C$ ≤ 1.25 D	1.25D $<C$ ≤ 1.5 D	1.5 D $<C$ ≤ 2 D	2 D $<C$ ≤ 3 D	3 D $<C$ ≤ 4 D	4 D $<C$ ≤ 5 D	$C > 5$ D
Pre	%	16.5	30.8	17.6	8.8	6.6	6.0	6.0	4.4	1.6	1.1	0.5
	n	30	56	32	16	12	11	11	8	3	2	1
1 week	%	51.6	24.7	14.8	4.9	1.6	0.5	1.1	0.5	0.0	0.0	0.0
	n	94	45	27	9	3	1	2	1	0	0	0
1 month	%	52.7	26.4	10.4	4.9	1.6	3.3	0.5	0.0	0.0	0.0	0.0
	n	96	48	19	9	3	6	1	0	0	0	0
3 months	%	54.4	23.6	9.3	7.7	3.3	1.1	0.5	0.0	0.0	0.0	0.0
	n	99	43	17	14	6	2	1	0	0	0	0
6 months	%	56.6	23.6	9.9	3.3	3.3	1.6	1.1	0.5	0.0	0.0	0.0
	n	103	43	18	6	6	3	2	1	0	0	0

Modified after Kunert et al. [13]
Distribution of astigmatism at appropriate follow-up intervals in 182 eyes

The undercorrection seemed to develop until 1 month and showed negligible variation at 1 month and thereafter. Looking at the data in more detail, there was a slight overcorrection in the low astigmatism group (0.5 D) and an undercorrection in higher astigmatism. In the range 1–3 D, the correction index was 0.87 and 0.93.

The corrected distance visual acuity (CDVA) at 6-month follow-up turned out that 96 % of the eyes had a CDVA of 20/20 or better and no eye has a CDVA worse than 20/32. Fifty-one percent of eyes had an unchanged corrected distance visual acuity, 33 % showed a gain of one line and 3 % a gain of two lines. Ten percent had lost one line, 2 % had lost two lines and 0.5 % (one eye) showed a loss of more than two lines of corrected distance visual acuity. In this study the old 200 kHz VisuMax® femtosecond laser was used for all procedures and all eyes had the flap lifted for the removal of the lenticule.

A number of changes took place after this study – the 500 kHz VisuMax® femtosecond laser entered the market, and according to the results of Kunert, an adjustment of the nomogram was added to the software. Furthermore flapless ReLEx® SMILE replaced ReLEx® FLEx as a mainstream procedure. Since corneal flap making has been reported to induce astigmatism [7], the presence (in ReLEx-FLEx) or absence (in ReLEx® SMILE) of a flap could affect astigmatic outcomes after surgery. To the best of our knowledge, no study has been published directly comparing the two techniques.

Ivarsen recently published results of ReLEx® SMILE treatments reporting an undercorrection with increased errors in treatment in higher astigmatism (see also Chap. 9) [15]. There is a range in the distribution of preoperative astigmatism (Kunert: −0.25 to −6.00 D vs. −1.00 to −2.75 D) in these two studies, in the surgical technique and in the repetition rate of the femtosecond laser (200 kHz vs. 500 kHz). The Huang study was published in 2000 and used microkeratome-created flaps. With today's femtosecond technology, it is possible to create thinner and more uniform flaps, and this might have resolved the astigmatism induction issue. A number of studies looking at higher-order aberration induction (HOA) by flap creation alone found only a small induction and not astigmatism. The induction of HOA in ReLEx® FLEx and ReLEx® SMILE was reported to be very similar [16, 17], and since the lenticule resection algorithms are identical for both techniques, a study to compare astigmatism induction would need a large sample size for statistical power. From a safety perspective, an undercorrection is an advantage for an early study because it is much easier to correct a postoperative myopic undercorrection than a hyperopic shift. It is likely that with gained experience the surgeons will be encouraged to more fully correct the cylinders by using suitable nomograms.

One possible reason for the observed undercorrection could be cyclotorsion. Prakash et al. reported that iris registration with eye tracking in LASIK gave better astigmatic results [18]. Kunerts analysis gave no evidence for cyclotorsion, because there was a nearly symmetrical variation in X and Y direction in the plots. Moreover, this was seen with and without left eye transformation. In the current stage iris registration is not available for the ReLEx procedure. The current software does not have any tools to adjust the axis of the entire resection profile (after the suction is applied) either. While some surgeons rotate the "contact glass" after the suction, if there is an evidence of cyclorotation, the manufacturer does not recommend this manoeuvre. Prior to the initiation of laser treatment, the laser scans the undersurface of the contact glass as a reference plane. A manual rotation of the contact glass might lead to an incorrect reference plane and jeopardize the accuracy of the calculated profile. Thus, currently the authors recommend to properly place patient's head and, if there is a cyclorotation, to release suction and reapply after head adjustment. Furthermore results might be improved by using larger transition zones.

In summary there is evidence that ReLEx® is a successful procedure for correcting myopic astigmatism. Although the results are good, future studies should focus on further improvement of astigmatic correction through nomograms, iris registration and optimized transition zones and the application of ReLEx® procedure.

References

1. Olsen T (1986) On the calculation of power from the curvature of the cornea. Br J Ophthalmol 70:152–154
2. Howland HC, Sayles N (1984) Photorefractive measurements of astigmatism in infants and young children. Invest Ophthalmol Vis Sci 25:93–102
3. Abrahamsson M, Fabian G, Sjorstrand J (1988) Changes in astigmatism between the ages of 1 and 4 years: a longitudinal study. Br J Ophthalmol 72:145–149
4. Saunders KJ (1995) Early refractive development in humans. Surv Ophthalmol 40:207–216
5. Thornton SP (1990) Astigmatic keratotomy: a review of basic concepts with case reports. J Cataract Refract Surg 16:430–435
6. Bailey MD, Zadnik K (2007) Outcomes of LASIK for myopia with FDA-approved lasers. Cornea 26:246–254
7. Huang D, Sur S, Seffo F, Meisler DM, Krueger RR (2000) Surgically-induced astigmatism after laser in situ keratomileusis for spherical myopia. J Refract Surg 16:515–518
8. Blum M, Kunert K, Schröder M, Sekundo W (2010) Femtosecond lenticule extraction for the correction of myopia: preliminary 6-month results. Graefes Arch Clin Exp Ophthalmol 248:1019–1027
9. Blum M, Kunert KS, Engelbrecht C, Dawczynski J, Sekundo W (2010) Femtosecond lenticule extraction (FLEx) – results after 12 months in myopic astigmatism. Klin Monbl Augenheilkd 227:961–965

10. Sekundo W, Kunert KS, Blum M (2011) Small incision corneal refractive surgery using the small incision lenticule extraction (SMILE) procedure for the correction of myopia and myopic astigmatism: results of a 6 month prospective study. Br J Ophthalmol 95:335–339
11. Shah R, Shah S (2011) Effect of scanning patterns on the results of femtosecond laser lenticule extraction refractive surgery. J Cataract Refract Surg 37:1636–1647
12. Blum M, Flach A, Kunert KS, Sekundo W (2014) Five-year results of refractive lenticule extraction. J Cataract Refract Surg 40:1425–1429
13. Kunert KS, Russmann C, Blum M, Sluyterman van Langenweyde G (2013) Vector analysis of myopic astigmatism corrected by femtosecond refractive lenticule extraction. J Cataract Refract Surg 39:759–769
14. Eydelman MB, Drum B, Holladay J, Hilmantel G, Kezirian G, Durrie D, Stulting RD, Sanders D, Wong B (2006) Standardized analyses of correction of astigmatism by laser systems that reshape the cornea. J Refract Surg 22:81–95
15. Ivarsen A, Hjortdal J (2014) Correction of myopic astigmatism with small lenticule extraction. J Refract Surg 30:240–247
16. Gertnere J, Solomatin I, Sekundo W (2013) Refractive lenticule extraction (ReLEx flex) and wavefront-optimized Femto-LASIK: comparison of contrast sensitivity and high-order aberrations at 1 year. Graefes Arch Clin Exp Ophthalmol 251:1437–1442
17. Sekundo W, Gertnere J, Bertelmann T, Solomatin I (2014) One-year refractive results, contrast sensitivity, high-order aberrations and complications after myopic small-incision lenticule extraction (ReLEx SMILE). Graefes Arch Clin Exp Ophthalmol 252:837–843
18. Prakash G, Agrawal A, Ashok Kumar D, Jacob S, Agrawal A (2011) Comparison of laser in situ keratomileusis for astigmatism without iris registration, with iris registration, and with iris registration-assisted dynamic eye tracking. J Cataract Refract Surg 37:574–581

Clinical Results in High Myopia

9

Anders Ivarsen and Jesper Hjortdal

Contents

Correction of high myopia has been attempted since the early days of keratorefractive surgery. Already in the 1950s, Barraquer developed keratomileusis as a lamellar treatment of very high refractive errors [20]. Barraquer's approach was widely acknowledged, but keratomileusis never reached widespread use due to highly variable outcomes and a technically demanding procedure. Later, in the 1970s Fyodorov advanced the use of radial incisions that were subsequently used to correct up to more than −10 diopters (D) of myopia [3]. In contrast to the complicated lamellar approaches, radial keratotomy was easily performed and became widely adopted. Still, results were unpredictable with long-term refractive instability as a severe complication [13].

The advent of the excimer laser in the late 1980s heralded a new age in keratorefractive surgery, with surface ablation procedures such as photorefractive keratectomy (PRK), and later the flap-based laser in situ keratomileusis (LASIK). At an early stage, attempts to correct myopia of more than −20 D were performed with PRK or LASIK [4, 11]; however, both procedures were found to have significant

A. Ivarsen, PhD (✉) • J. Hjortdal, DMSc
Department of Ophthalmology, Aarhus University Hospital, Aarhus, Denmark
e-mail: ai@dadlnet.dk; jesper.hjortdal@dadlnet.dk

© Springer International Publishing Switzerland 2015
W. Sekundo (ed.), *Small Incision Lenticule Extraction (SMILE):*
Principles, Techniques, Complication Management, and Future Concepts,
DOI 10.1007/978-3-319-18530-9_9

complications with high myopic corrections. Thus, several factors were realized to influence the precision of the photoablative procedure, including corneal hydration, room humidity, patient age, parallax error, and laser fluency [1, 25], all causing reduced predictability with higher attempted correction. In surface ablation procedures, correction of high myopia was also found to cause more postoperative wound healing increasing the risk of stromal haze formation and reduced long-term stability of the obtained refractive correction [23]. In LASIK, high corrections were associated with an increased risk of iatrogenic keratectasia [15, 19]. Still, PRK and LASIK represent highly successful surgical procedures due to excellent patient satisfaction, high precision, and a very good safety, but today PRK is predominantly recommended for correction of low degrees of myopia and LASIK for myopia of less than −8 to −10 D.

Within the last 5 years, femtosecond laser-based refractive lenticule extraction using the VisuMax (Carl Zeiss Meditec) laser platform has emerged as the most recent development in keratorefractive surgery, with small incision lenticule extraction (SMILE) as the latest evolutionary step [17, 18, 24]. In SMILE, the cutting of a lenticule within the intact corneal stroma has removed many of the variable factors known from excimer-based procedures. Furthermore, in SMILE most of the anterior stromal lamellae are left intact, and it has been suggested that the biomechanical impact is less in SMILE than in other keratorefractive procedures [16], indicating that it might be safe to attempt correction of high refractive errors. However, biomechanical studies on SMILE-treated corneas using the Ocular Response Analyzer or Scheimpflug-based imaging (Corvis ST) has not found any consistent differences from LASIK [21, 26], and for safety reasons the VisuMax laser does not allow correction of more than −10 D at present.

Most studies on clinical outcome after SMILE consider correction of low to moderate myopia; however, in the present chapter, the clinical outcomes after SMILE for myopia of −6 D or more are reviewed.

9.1   Refractive Outcome

Overall, the refractive predictability of SMILE for correction of high myopia has been reported to be very good (Table 9.1); however, so far most published studies in highly myopic eyes have had only 3 or 6 months follow-up. In a report of 670 eyes treated with SMILE for an average of −7.19 ± 1.30 D, the mean error in spherical equivalent refraction 3 months after surgery was −0.25 ± 0.44 D, with 80 % of eyes being within ±0.50 D and 94 % within ±1.0 D [6]. In an extension of the same study, we found a similar mean error of −0.15 ± 0.50 D in 1,574 eyes, with 77 % of eyes being within ±0.50 D and 95 % within ±1.0 D [7]. Other papers with fewer patients have all found similar outcomes with 77–93 % of eyes being within ±0.50 D, 3–6 months after SMILE for high myopia [10, 22, 24, 27]. In one paper, 1-year refractive data were reported after SMILE for an average myopia of −5.84 D. Although technically not high myopia, this study found 88 % of the treated eyes to be within ±0.50 D after 12 months, with an average overcorrection of 0.10 ± 0.37 D [2].

Table 9.1 Overview of studies on SMILE in high myopia reporting preoperative refraction, refractive outcome, visual outcome, and safety

	Study method	Preop. Sph.eq. refraction (D)	N (eyes)	Follow-up (months)	Refractive outcome	Regression	Visual outcome	2-line loss in CDVA
Hjortdal et al. [6]	Prospective	−7.19±1.30	670	3	80 % within ±0.5 D	Not reported	84 % UDVA ≥20/25	2.4 %
Vestergaard et al. [24]	Prospective	−7.18±1.57	279	3	77 % within ±0.5 D	0.15 D	73 % UDVA ≥20/25	0.4 %
Ivarsen et al. [7]	Prospective	−7.25±1.84	1,574	3	77 % within ±0.5 D	Not reported	Not reported	1.5 %
Zhao et al. [27]	Prospective	−6.67±1.43	54	6	93 % within ±0.5 D	None	98 % UDVA ≥20/20	None
Vestergaard et al. [22]	Prospective	−7.56±1.11	34	6	88 % within ±0.5 D	None	83 % UDVA ≥20/25	None
Kim et al. [10]	Prospective	−6.18±1.67	293	6	86 % within ±0.5 D	None	98 % UDVA ≥20/25	0.3 %
Ang et al. [2]	Prospective	−5.84±2.12[a]	35	12	88 % within ±0.5 D	None	77 % UDVA ≥20/20	None

Corrected distance visual acuity (*CDVA*), uncorrected distance visual acuity (*UDVA*)

[a]Study on moderate myopia included since it is the only publication on 12-month data

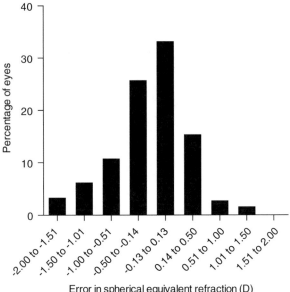

Fig. 9.1 Error in spherical equivalent refraction given as the percentage of eyes obtaining the specified refraction 3 years after SMILE for high myopia ($n = 174$)

Error in spherical equivalent refraction (D)

In addition, we recently evaluated 174 eyes 3 years after SMILE for an average myopia of -7.30 ± 1.35 D and found a mean refractive error of -0.19 ± 1.04 D, with 75 % of eyes being within ± 0.50 D and 89 % within ± 1.0 D (Fig. 9.1).

The long-term refractive stability after SMILE for correction of high myopia has not been extensively investigated. However, in one study on 279 eyes, refraction was found to be stable from 1 to 3 months after surgery, although a minor regression of -0.15 D was observed during the first month [24]. Another study on 54 eyes found no regression during the first 6 months after surgery [27], and similarly the study on SMILE for an average of -5.84 D found no significant changes in refraction from 1 to 12 months after surgery [2]. In our recent evaluation 3 years after SMILE for high myopia, we also found no significant refractive regression in 84 eyes from 1 month to 3 years after surgery (Fig. 9.2).

The refractive predictability in combined high myopia and astigmatism represents a particular challenge, but overall 77 % of 775 eyes have been reported to be within ±0.50 D of the attempted spherical equivalent refraction after 3 months, irrespective of the attempted astigmatic correction [8]. Nevertheless, increasing undercorrection of the astigmatic component was observed with higher attempted corrections at an average of 16 % per diopter.

Interestingly, the predictability after SMILE has been found to be unrelated to the degree of the attempted myopic correction [6]. This stands in contrast to excimer-based treatments where corneal hydration, room humidity, patient age, parallax error, and laser fluency affect the ablative procedure [1, 25], giving rise to decreasing precision with increasing myopic correction. Furthermore, preoperative corneal

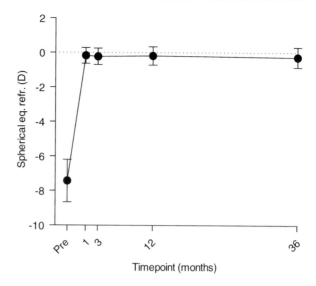

Fig. 9.2 Mean error in spherical equivalent refraction of 84 eyes from 1 month to 3 years after SMILE for high myopia

power, patient age, and gender have been found to have very limited impact on the refractive outcome after SMILE [6, 10].

9.2   Visual Outcome

In the few studies reporting visual outcome after SMILE for high myopia, 73–100 % of patients had an uncorrected distance visual acuity (UDVA) of 20/25 or better 3–6 months after surgery (Table 9.1). Ang et al. similarly reported 77 % of patients to have an UDVA of 20/20 or better 12 months after correction for an average of −5.84 D [2]. In our recent 3-year evaluation of SMILE for an average of −7.30 ± 1.35 D, we found an UDVA of 20/25 or better in 82 % of 174 eyes (Fig. 9.3).

The efficacy index 3 months after SMILE (postoperative UDVA/preoperative CDVA) was reported to be 0.90 ± 0.25 in a prospective study of 670 eyes, indicating that a patient on average can expect a postoperative UDVA of 90 % of their preoperative CDVA [6].

Overall the results after SMILE seem to be on par with those after FS-LASIK in high myopic corrections [28].

9.3   Higher Order Aberrations

In excimer laser surgery it is well established that higher myopic corrections induce more high-order aberrations (HOAs) [14]. Large amounts of HOAs reduce the visual performance under poor lighting conditions and contribute to night vision

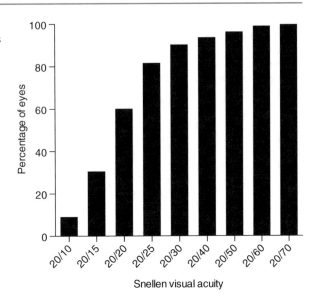

Fig. 9.3 Uncorrected distance visual acuity 3 years after SMILE for high myopia in 149 eyes with an attempted postoperative refraction of ±0.25 D

disturbances after refractive surgery. In two studies, SMILE has been found to induce less HOAs than FS-LASIK when correcting low to moderate myopia [5, 12]. However, the induced HOAs after high myopic correction have not yet been systematically investigated, and it remains to be determined whether SMILE offers any advantage over excimer laser procedures with respect to the postoperative aberrations.

9.4   Safety of High Myopic Corrections

In refractive surgery, the overall safety may be assessed by the induced change in corrected distance visual acuity (CDVA). In general, loss or gain of two or more lines on the Snellen visual acuity card is considered to be significant and noticeable for the patient.

Most of the current studies on SMILE for high myopia are too small to properly evaluate the safety of the procedure, but the frequency of a 2-line loss in CDVA has been reported to lie between 0 and 2.4 % in high myopic corrections (Table 9.1). In one study, 0.3 % of 293 eyes were reported to have a loss of 2 or more lines [10]. In contrast, a study by Hjortdal et al. of 670 eyes treated with SMILE for high myopia found a 2.4 % risk for a significant loss of CDVA [6]. Yet, in the same study, a safety index (CDVA before/CDVA after surgery) of 1.07 ± 0.22 was found, indicating that CDVA on average increased after surgery, as would be expected due to the image magnification induced by the myopic keratorefractive procedure.

Furthermore, in an evaluation of 1,574 SMILE procedures for high myopia we found CDVA to have improved with 2 or more lines in 3.4 % of eyes, whereas 1.5 % of eyes had experienced a loss of 2 or more lines [7]. However, all patients with a loss in visual acuity were re-evaluated after more than 1 year and were found to have recovered to within one line of their preoperative CDVA. The surgeon learning curve and laser settings were found to be important parameters for the postoperative visual recovery. Overall, the safety after SMILE for high myopia appears to be on par with that reported after FS-LASIK, although visual recovery may be prolonged in some patients.

A rare complication to SMILE may be development of postoperative irregular astigmatism with monocular ghost images that has been found in 6 out of 1,574 eyes treated for high myopia [7]. Topography-guided PRK has been reported to ameliorate symptoms in these patients, although mitomycin C should be used even in shallow excimer laser ablations to reduce the risk of postoperative haze development [9].

As of yet, no cases of postoperative ectasia have been reported after SMILE for high myopia.

Conclusion

Although the number of publications on SMILE for high myopic corrections is still relatively small, evidence is accumulating that the refractive and visual outcome after SMILE is as good as after FS-LASIK, with minimal to no postoperative refractive regression. Furthermore, studies on low to moderate myopic corrections indicate that SMILE induces less HOAs than excimer-based surgery. This is of particular interest in high myopia where the induction of HOAs is more pronounced in excimer-based procedures.

However, in the context of high myopic corrections, the most interesting aspect of SMILE may be the minimal impact on the anterior stroma. Due to the intact anterior stromal lamellae, the cornea has been suggested to be stronger after SMILE than after excimer-based treatments, in theory reducing the risk of iatrogenic keratectasia. Thus, very high myopic corrections might be safe, although the biomechanical advantage of SMILE has proven elusive and has not yet been clinically confirmed.

In its current state, SMILE has been shown to be a reliable, efficient, and safe procedure for high myopic corrections, and now 3-year data is gradually becoming available. Still, it is of utmost interest to follow the outcomes and evolution of SMILE for high myopic corrections over the coming years.

References

1. Ang E, Couper T, Dirani M et al (2009) Outcomes of laser refractive surgery for myopia. J Cataract Refract Surg 35(5):921–933
2. Ang M, Mehta J, Chan C et al (2014) Refractive lenticule extraction: transition and comparison of 3 surgical techniques. J Cataract Refract Surg 40(9):1415–1424
3. Bores L, Myers W, Cowden J (1981) Radial keratotomy: an analysis of the American experience. Ann Ophthalmol 13(8):941–948
4. Fyodorov S, Semyonov A, Magaramov M et al (1993) PRK using an absorbing cell delivery system for correction of myopia from 4 to 26 D in 3251 eyes. Refract Corneal Surg 9(2 Suppl):S123–S124
5. Ganesh S, Gupta R (2014) Comparison of visual and refractive outcomes following femtosecond laser- assisted lasik with smile in patients with myopia or myopic astigmatism. J Refract Surg 30(9):590–596

6. Hjortdal J, Vestergaard A, Ivarsen A et al (2012) Predictors for the outcome of small-incision lenticule extraction for Myopia. J Refract Surg 28(12):865–871
7. Ivarsen A, Asp S, Hjortdal J (2014) Safety and complications of more than 1500 small-incision lenticule extraction procedures. Ophthalmology 121(4):822–828
8. Ivarsen A, Hjortdal J (2014) Correction of myopic astigmatism with small incision lenticule extraction. J Refract Surg 30(4):240–247
9. Ivarsen A, Hjortdal J (2014) Topography-guided photorefractive keratectomy for irregular astigmatism after small incision lenticule extraction. J Refract Surg 30(6):429–432
10. Kim J, Hwang H, Mun S et al (2014) Efficacy, predictability, and safety of small incision lenticule extraction: 6-months prospective cohort study. BMC Ophthalmol 14:117
11. Knorz M, Liermann A, Seiberth V et al (1996) Laser in situ keratomileusis to correct myopia of −6.00 to −29.00 diopters. J Refract Surg 12(5):575–584
12. Lin F, Xu Y, Yang Y (2014) Comparison of the visual results after SMILE and femtosecond laser-assisted LASIK for myopia. J Refract Surg 39(4):248–254
13. McDonnell P, Nizam A, Lynn M et al (1996) Morning-to-evening change in refraction, corneal curvature, and visual acuity 11 years after radial keratotomy in the prospective evaluation of radial keratotomy study. The PERK Study Group. Ophthalmology 103(2):233–239
14. Oshika T, Miyata K, Tokunaga T et al (2002) Higher order wavefront aberrations of cornea and magnitude of refractive correction in laser in situ keratomileusis. Ophthalmology 109(6):1154–1158
15. Rad A, Jabbervand M, Saifi N (2004) Progressive keratectasia after laser in situ keratomileusis. J Refract Surg 20(5 Suppl):S718–S722
16. Reinstein D, Archer T, Randleman J (2013) Mathematical model to compare the relative tensile strength of the cornea after PRK, LASIK, and small incision lenticule extraction. J Refract Surg 29(7):454–460
17. Sekundo W, Kunert K, Russmann C et al (2008) First efficacy and safety study of femtosecond lenticule extraction for the correction of myopi: six month results. J Cataract Refract Surg 34(9):1513–1520
18. Shah R, Shah S, Sengupta S (2011) Results of small incision lenticule extraction: All-in-one femtosecond laser refractive surgery. J Cataract Refract Surg 37:127–37
19. Spadea L, Palmieri G, Mosca L et al (2002) Iatrogenic keratectasia following laser in situ keratomileusis. J Refract Surg 18(4):475–480
20. Swinger C, Barraquer J (1981) Keratophakia and keratomileusis–clinical results. Ophthalmology 88(8):709–715
21. Vestergaard A, Grauslund J, Ivarsen A et al (2014) Central Corneal Sublayer Pachymetry and Biomechanical Properties After Refractive Femtosecond Lenticule Extraction. J Refract Surg 30(2):102–108
22. Vestergaard A, Grauslund J, Ivarsen A et al (2014) Efficacy, safety, predictability, contrast sensitivity, and aberrations after femtosecond laser lenticule extraction. J Cataract Refract Surg 40(3):403–411
23. Vestergaard A, Hjortdal J, Ivarsen A et al (2013) Long-term outcomes of photorefractive keratectomy for low to high myopia: 13 to 19 years of follow-up. J Refract Surg 29(5):312–319
24. Vestergaard A, Ivarsen A, Asp S et al (2012) Small-incision lenticule extraction for moderate to high myopia: Predictability, safety, and patient satisfaction. J Cataract Refract Surg 38(11):2003–2010
25. Walter K, Stevensen A (2004) Effect of environmental factors on myopic LASIK enhancement rates. J Cataract Refract Surg 30(4):798–803
26. Wang D, Liu M, Chen Y et al (2014) Differences in the Corneal Biomechanical Changes After SMILE and LASIK. J Refract Surg 30(10):702–707
27. Zhao J, Yao P, Chen Z et al (2013) The Morphology of Corneal Cap and Its Relation to Refractive Outcomes in Femtosecond Laser Small Incision Lenticule Extraction (SMILE) with Anterior Segment Optical Coherence Tomography Observation. PLoS One 8(8), e70208
28. Zhao L, Zhu H, Li L (2014) Laser-assisted subepithelial keratectomy versus laser in situ keratomileusis in myopia: a systematic review and meta-analysis. ISRN Ophthalmol:672146. doi: 10.1155/2014/672146

Complications After SMILE and Its Management Including Re-treatment Techniques

10

Rupal Shah

Contents

Financial Disclosure The author is a consultant for Carl Zeiss Meditec AG and receives study and travel support from Carl Zeiss Meditec AG

Electronic supplementary material The online version of this chapter (doi:10.1007/978-3-319-18530-9_10) contains supplementary material, which is available to authorized users.

R. Shah, MS
New Vision Laser Centers-Centre for Sight, Mumbai, India
e-mail: rupal@newvisionindia.com

© Springer International Publishing Switzerland 2015
W. Sekundo (ed.), *Small Incision Lenticule Extraction (SMILE): Principles, Techniques, Complication Management, and Future Concepts*, DOI 10.1007/978-3-319-18530-9_10

Any surgery has some potential complications. Awareness of these can help to develop strategies to avoid them or – if they happen – to react appropriately. If the surgeon is aware of potential complications, and ways to mitigate them or recover from them, it is easy to react quickly during and after surgery. Moreover, relative to LASIK or Femto-LASIK, the SMILE procedure requires more surgical dexterity and skill. This can lead to complications from which it is not easy to recover. In the present chapter we give a short overview of the hitherto known complications and our subjective opinion on their management. It is obvious that despite our best efforts, this chapter cannot raise a claim to cover all the complications or to give the best possible solutions. Rather, it should be treated as a useful guide and starting point.

10.1   Intraoperative Complications

There are a number of intraoperative complications that can occur during the SMILE procedure. Some of these include:

(a) A suction loss wherein the contact glass and cornea become detached during the procedure and the procedure is then aborted by the laser
(b) During the lenticule separation process, while trying to separate the anterior lenticule surface from the overlying cornea, the wrong cleavage plane is selected by the surgeon, and the posterior part of the lenticule is separated instead. In such a situation, the lenticule sticks to the undersurface of the corneal cap, with resultant difficulty in separating and removing the lenticule.
(c) Incomplete removal of the lenticule or tearing of only a part of the lenticule
(d) Tearing of the corneal cap at the incision edge
(e) Creation of a wrong deeper dissection plane (so-called via falsa) by forceful manual dissection

In our opinion, with the exception of (e), none of these are vision threatening and, if managed well, allow the procedure to be completed with a normal result.

10.1.1 Suction Loss Wherein the Contact Glass and the Cornea Become Detached During the Laser Firing Procedure

This can happen due to several reasons:

(a) Most commonly, the patient squeezes the eye or moves suddenly.
(b) There could be fluid ingress between the suction ports of the contact glass and the cornea.
(c) Gas bubble migration and subsequent compressive forces against the contact glass.

In this situation, the VisuMax® automatically goes into a specific mode, based on the stage of the procedure at which the suction loss occurred.

In case the suction loss occurs during the *first pass* of the laser (i.e., the pass which defines the posterior surface of the lenticule), the user is *not* given the option to complete the procedure and is asked to convert the procedure into a Femto-LASIK procedure. The user can do this in the same surgical session (Video 10.1). In our experience, it is also possible to postpone the procedure for a few minutes or days and then complete the procedure from scratch (Video 10.2). However, if one decides to redo SMILE some time later, a different depth of the lenticule's bottom may be considered in order to avoid entering of the old incision. This measure may be of value, since one might not want the existing cleavage plane to interact with the new cleavage plane being created for the posterior surface of the lenticule in an unpredictable fashion.

If the suction loss occurs at any other stage during the laser firing procedure, the laser allows the option of completing the procedure in the same surgical session after re-docking of the contact glass (Videos 10.3 and 10.4). The general challenge in this situation is re-docking of the contact glass interface to the eye while still retaining the original centration. This is because the pupil is obscured by the gas bubbles from the earlier pass(es). It is preferable to use the same contact glass, so that the foot prints of the contact glass match. Proper centration during re-docking is extremely important. Once re-docking is completed, depending on the stage at which suction loss occurs, the laser repeats both femtosecond passes, only the "cap" pass or only the side cut incision. The lenticule separation and removal is then carried out as usual.

Sharma and Vadavalli [1] reported a case of an eye of an uncooperative patient where there was suction loss during the "cap" cut (i.e., when more than 90 % of the procedure was completed). The surgeon attempted to re-dock and repeat the procedure. Unfortunately, there was another suction loss, and the procedure was abandoned. The surgeon then successfully completed a Femto-LASIK flap, with the same thickness as the original "cap."

10.1.2 During Lenticule Separation, the Lenticule Sticking to the Undersurface of the Cap

The second intraoperative complication generally observed is that while trying to separate the anterior lenticule surface from the overlying cornea (which is the first step in the lenticule separation procedure), the wrong plane is selected by the surgeon, and the posterior part of the lenticule is separated instead. In this case, the lenticule remains stuck on the undersurface of the flap, rather than on the stromal bed.

This situation offers a surgical challenge, because without the anchor of the posterior cornea, trying to enter the anterior cleavage plane for separation is a difficult exercise.

Once the problem is recognized, then it is still, in our opinion, possible to separate and remove the lenticule. In my preferred technique, I use the hook end of the double-sided intralase spatula to try and gently scrape a small edge of the lenticule from the anterior "cap." Instead of attempting this at center of the incision, I try and do this at the sides of the incision. Once a small edge is available, I use a Shah SMILE forceps to hold the edge and peel off a little more of the lenticule. Once sufficient space is available, I insert the separation spatula and separate and remove the lenticule in the usual way. If the entering incision is too small, one can enlarge it slightly along the cap border using a preset diamond knife or even an MVR blade.

Recently, some rescue instruments have been developed by the Mehta group in Singapore (also see Chap. 5) for dealing with this complication, which are in the nature of a rake, wedge, or hook. Using these instruments, the surgeon can go to the edge of the lenticule at the inferior part of the cornea and try to separate the lenticule from that end and then use the instrument to progressively remove the lenticule along its entire circumferential edge (Videos 10.5, 10.6, and 10.7).

10.1.3 Tearing of the Lenticule and/or Lenticule Tags Being Left Behind While Doing the Lenticule Separation and Removal

Tearing of the lenticule can occur if it is a thin lenticule or the laser separation is not optimal (because of severe opaque bubble layer or corneal opacities or a fiber or other foreign matter between the contact glass and the cornea). In this case, while attempting the separation, the lenticule gets torn.

A surgeon can also inadvertently leave some lenticule tags behind, especially at the edges.

If some portion of the lenticule remains behind, it can result in irregular astigmatism and an unacceptable outcome.

To prevent this from happening, it is best to do a complete separation in the first instance. It is best to use the spatula to completely separate the lenticule from both surfaces, along the entire circumference. It is best *not* to attempt to partially separate the lenticule and then grasp the lenticule with a forceps and then pull or tug at the unseparated portions. This increases the risk of lenticule tearing and of tags being left behind.

When the surgeon is in doubt about the lenticule tearing or of tags being left behind, it is best to uncurl the lenticule on the epithelial surface of the cornea after removing it and check to see if its size matches the original edge of the laser separation along its entire diameter.

In case it is suspected that some lenticule tags have been left behind, then it is possible, even at a later date, to go in from the same incision site and remove the tags.

10.1.4 Tearing of the Corneal Cap at the Incision Edge

With the trend towards smaller and smaller side cut incisions, with some surgeons even using only 1.5 mm incisions, it is possible to tear the corneal cap at the edges of the incision.

In our opinion, if the tear is small and outside the pupillary area, it has no adverse outcome other than a small scar. If the tear is large, one can align the anterior surface properly and put a bandage contact lens on. Usually it heals with a very faint line only. However, there is a higher risk of epithelial ingrowth (see below) (Fig. 10.1). It is best to prevent such a tear, however. The surgeon should only attempt to use an incision size commensurate with their experience and surgical dexterity.

10.1.5 Gas Breakthrough from One Laser Plane into the Other Plane

This absolutely exceptional complication was witnessed only once in a case referred for a second opinion. Indeed, it is almost impossible to recognize it during the scan and, if suspected, should be left alone and not dissected. The reason is lenticule which is too thin. Thus, a minimum lenticule central thickness of 50 μm is recommended. For further details, please see Chap. 7.

10.1.6 Forceful Dissection of the Wrong Plane Deeper than the Cleavage Plane Created by the Laser

This extremely rare complication was referred to us twice for a second opinion. In both cases the surgeon was novel to the procedure. This complication, in our view, is a result of a totally improper handling of the tissue. Little resistance to the dissection spatula is normal. However, if the surgeon encounters severe resistance reminiscent of lamellar keratoplasty, the procedure should be abandoned and no tissue removed from within the cornea. Otherwise a permanent damage will occur, relievable only by a lamellar anterior/inter-pocket/deep anterior lamellar keratoplasty.

10.2 Postoperative Complications After SMILE

10.2.1 Epithelial Ingrowth

Sometimes epithelial ingrowth can be observed, after SMILE. Unlike with LASIK, where ablation of the hinge can sometimes result in a path for the epithelium to encroach under the flap, in SMILE, it is usually an isolated nest of cells. They can either be left alone, if the nest is silent, or it can be scraped off by entering with an epithelial scraper from the original incision (Fig. 10.1).

10.2.2 Irregular Astigmatism Consequent to Decentration

Sometimes, if the docking procedure is not correct, it can result in decentration of the treatment and consequent irregular astigmatism and/or induction of aberrations, such as coma.

Fig. 10.1 The superior incision had an anticlockwise radial tear with a subsequent epithelial ingrowth. One year after surgery the ingrowth remained stationary without any effect on visual performance of the eye (Photograph by W. Sekundo)

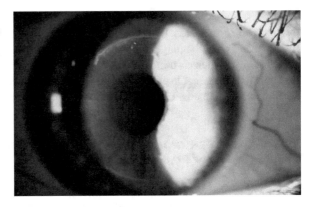

In our opinion, it is best to prevent this complication. Following the proper docking procedure is essential. We also find it useful to switch to infrared illumination for a brief period after docking (and before initiating the laser pass), to verify that the pupil dilates around the center of the contact glass.

In case decentration occurs, and it is visually significant, then it is best to perform a topography-guided excimer laser correction using PRK [2], keeping in mind the cap thickness.

10.2.3 Other Postoperative Complications

In some cases, a fine scarring is observed at the cap edge or the lenticule edge. However, this is outside the pupillary zone and is visually nonsignificant. Some patients, especially chronic contact lens users before the procedure, experience dry eyes after the procedure. We have also observed a few cases of a fine interface haze several months after the procedure. In the majority of cases it is not visually significant. Since the haze is sometimes related to ease of dissection, some surgeons increase and prolong their steroid regimen in cases of difficult dissection. We also observed a positive effect of fluoromet021alone drops in cases of an increased haze 2 months after surgery. If a longer course of steroids is not desired, 1 % cyclosporin A (CSA) eye drops twice daily for several months helps to reverse the course.

Due to a geometrical mismatch between the undersurface of the cap and the stromal bed after lenticule removal, some microstriae, named "Bowman's layer microdistortions" (BLMD), have been described particularly after highly myopic SMILE [3]. In the majority of cases these microfolds are smoothed out by the epithelium as time goes by. If desired, an early intervention with pressurized flushing of the pocket can be attempted (B. Meyer, personal communication). Prior to such radical measures an anterior high-resolution OCT scan is of value. To prevent

Fig. 10.2 An epithelial abrasion around the entering incision as shown in this example is usually fully epithelialized within 24 h. However, the surgeon should carefully observe the interface for the development of localized DLK and increase topical steroids, if necessary (Photograph by W. Sekundo)

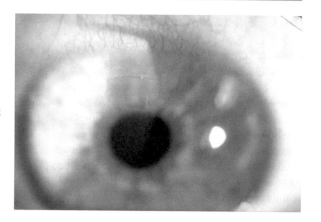

visually significant folds in the optical zone, one is advised to gently massage the cap centrifugally as suggested by Reinstein et al. [4].

Unlike in FS-Lasik surgery sterile keratitis is extremely rare. Severe inflammation has also been observed after the procedure, especially if (a) the energy settings of the laser are too high or (b) one has a large periincisional epithelial abrasion (Fig. 10.2) or even an intraoperative epithelial slough off (usually in eyes with epithelial basement membrane dystrophy) or (c) some debris were left behind in the pocket. Usually this resolves with steriods and/or flushing of the debris with no visual significance. An exception is a secondary interlamellar keratitis due to steroid-induced IOP rise, as described by Shimizu. Here, flushing the pocket and discontinuation of steroids will resolve the problem.

Infection, like with any other procedure, can also occur and is probably best managed not only by topical medication, but also by pocket flushing and drug injection into the interface.

Lastly, like any corneal subtraction procedure, there is also risk of corneal ectasia. However, among LASIK, FS-LASIK, and SMILE, it would make sense that SMILE would have the lowest ectasia rate. Nevertheless, caution needs to be observed in making sure that corrections are not attempted that would make the cornea excessively thin. The reader is also referred to Chap. 21 describing an experimental procedure of combined SMILE and cross-linking.

10.2.4 Unknown Causes of Poor Visual Recovery

In very rare circumstances we see cases with perfect topographies, reasonable ocular surface, and nice appearance on anterior segment OCT but yet loss of two lines or more. We currently do not have an answer to what is the reason, but have had a positive experience with waiting over 1 year and supporting the corneal surface by both hyaluronic acid containing lubricants and CSA eye drops.

10.3   Enhancements After SMILE

Like any other refractive surgery procedure, there is likely to be the need for enhancements after the procedure. This can be because of a myopic drift several years after the procedure or because of a primary over- or undercorrection. This presents a peculiar problem after the SMILE procedure, because it does not offer the chance of lifting the flap and performing excimer laser reshaping, which is relatively easy after LASIK or the FLEx procedure. Enhancements after SMILE can be completed using excimer laser PRK; however, additional use of mitomycin C is recommended, even in very small corrections to prevent haze formation. We do not have experience with ultrathin flap Femto-LASIK in the cap or a second SMILE in a thick cap or below the original incision for performing enhancements, though some surgeons have done this successfully.

Recently, a new procedure, dubbed "CIRCLE" has been developed to convert the original SMILE cap into a complete flap, with a hinge and a 270–330° side cut incision. In the CIRCLE procedure, the femtosecond laser is used to create (a) an incision plane encircling the original "cap" cut as a lamellar ring and (b) a side cut with hinge around the new incision plane and (c) a "junction cut" which allows the original "cap" and the new incision plane to be part of one larger surface (Fig. 10.3). Riau et al. [5] investigated the use of four different patterns to create the above three cuts in rabbit eyes. They found the pattern (pattern D) which creates the lamellar ring at the same level as the original "cap" thickness to be the easiest to lift, even though all four patterns created a viable flap. In our own clinical experience in human eyes, the CIRCLE software is easy to use and reliably creates flaps which can be lifted easily to perform excimer laser reshaping after lifting the flap (Video 10.8).

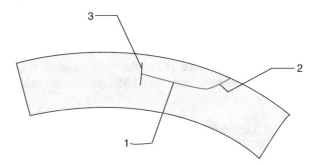

Fig. 10.3 A crosssectional view of the CIRCLE femtosecond incisions. A lamellar ring is created around the original "cap" cut, and in addition, a junction cut connected the cap to the lamellar ring, and a sidecut incision with hinge is provided

References

1. Sharma R, Vadavalli PK (2013) Implications and management of suction loss during refractive lenticule extraction (ReLEx). J Refract Surg 29(7):502–503
2. Ivarsen A, Hjordtal J (2014) Topography-guided photorefractive keratectomy for irregular astigmatism after small incision lenticule extraction. J Refract Surg 30(6):429–432
3. Yao P, Zhou J, Meiyan L, Shen Y, Dong Z, Zhou X (2013) Microdistortions in Bowman's layer following femtosecond laser small incision lenticule extraction observed by Fourier-Domain OCT. J Refract Surg 29(10):668–674
4. Reinstein DZ, Archer TJ, Gobbe M (2014) Small incision lenticule extraction (SMILE). History, fundamentals of a new refractive surgery technique and clinical outcomes. Eye Vis 1:3
5. Riau AK, Ang HP, Lwin NC, Chaurasia SS, Tan DT, Mehta JS (2013) Comparison of four different VisuMax circle patterns for flap creation after small incision lenticule extraction. J Refract Surg 29(4):236–244

Management of Laser Settings for Better SMILE Surgery

11

Bertram Meyer and Rainer Wiltfang

Contents

We started with ReLEx® SMILE, because the advantages of this refractive procedure were very convincing. This method seems to be safe and effective, independent of environmental conditions and corneal hydration and with a high level of biomechanical stability of the cornea postoperatively.

The biggest challenges we were faced with during the early days of SMILE were the delayed visual recovery during the first post-op days, the ideal way of enhancement, and the possible treatment range in the long term.

In this chapter we explain how we optimized the clinical settings to improve the clinical outcome for this treatment. Because the majority of newer VisuMax® lasers are equipped with the mode, where some adjustments can be made by the individual surgeon, this short chapter will explain the interaction between the energy and the spot size/track distance and provide the reader with understanding on how to further optimize his or her individual laser.

B. Meyer, MD (✉)
Eye Center (Augencentrum) Cologne, Josefstraße 14, 51143 Koeln, Germany
e-mail: Bertram.Meyer@t-online.de

R. Wiltfang, MD
Eye Center (Augencentrum) Cologne, Josefstraße 14, 51143 Koeln, Germany
e-mail: wiltfang@smileeyes.de

© Springer International Publishing Switzerland 2015
W. Sekundo (ed.), *Small Incision Lenticule Extraction (SMILE):*
Principles, Techniques, Complication Management, and Future Concepts,
DOI 10.1007/978-3-319-18530-9_11

First we defined the possible parameters that might influence and be responsible for delayed visual recovery. In our opinion there are two possible factors:

1. The level of energy per area (basically the fluency) and as a consequence thereof the development of gas bubbles following plasma development increase tissue compression. This in turn leads to an irregular surface seen as an abnormal topography.
2. Optimized spot and tracking spacing to reduce the roughness of the residual stroma and lenticule's surface.

The precision of tissue preparation both prior and during the cut is essential for accurate refractive outcomes. Preventing tissue distortion seems to be crucial.

To prevent tissue distortion prior to the cut, we take advantage of a curved contact glass and a very low corneal suction pressure, hence causing a minimum applanation in the central cornea (see Fig. 4.1).

Unlike in flap cutting where only one plane is produced by laser, the interaction between the two adjacent planes (the so-called refractive and non-refractive cut) is of utmost importance. Thus, the second goal was to get a smooth bubble layer during the first deeper cut, in order to prevent tissue distortion while doing the second cut.

Optical breakdown generates plasma and consequently gas bubbles are formed.

——— intended cut   ◯ single gas bubble

As a physiological principle, single gas bubbles join to form fewer, but bigger gas bubbles if they are close enough. These big bubbles are deforming the surrounding tissue.

Consequently the upper cut is created within this deformed tissue.

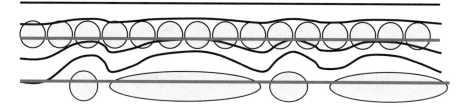

After tissue relaxation and absorption of the gas bubbles, the intended layer of the cut will deviate from the real cut. Extracting such a "deformed" lenticule would result in huge iatrogenic aberrations and in a lower quality of visual outcomes.

resulting real cut

To avoid this, the volume of gas bubbles must be kept as low as possible while the distance between the single bubbles should remain both small enough for an effective separation and still large enough for preventing tight junctions.

The first step to shorten the time between the laser cut between the two interfaces (the "bottom" and the "roof") in the central cornea (the optical zone) was achieved by Shah simply by changing the cut direction. This is the reason why the current scan direction is "spiral-in" followed by "spiral-out" [1].

We decided to go further: The goal was to find the best combination of energy levels and spot and tracking distances to enhance the cut quality and the ease of tissue separation.

In order to find the right management of laser settings, we started with basic research.

The first trials have been done on pig eyes to find out the limits of energy and spot distances:

Table 11.1 shows how to find outer limits for the three given variables. Please also note: VisuMax laser uses so-called index for laser energy settings. For the purpose of simplicity we keep this "index" as a unit VisuMax users are used to. However, one can keep in mind that one index unit approximately corresponds to 5 nJ.

Table 11.1 3 groups of different energy settings per area on pig eyes

ID	Sphere/lenticule thickness	Flap energy/lenticule energy	Track distance/spot distance (μm)
5	−5 D/96 μm	Index* 60	2.0/2.0
6	−10 D/166 μm	Index 60	2.0/2.0
11	−5 D/96 μm	Index 60	3.5/3.5
12	−10 D/166 μm	Index 60	3.5/3.5
13	−5 D/96 μm	Index 22	5.0/5.0
14	−10 D/166 μm	Index 22	5.0/5.0

*1 index unit is approx. 5nJ (e.g. index 60 = 300nJ)

With high energy (index 60) and small spot and tracking distance (2.0 or 3.5 μ), we found stromal ring-shaped structures.

With low energy (index 22) and big spot and tracking distance (5.0 μ), there was no way for a controlled tissue separation anymore.

The best combination of energy level and spot and tracking distance regarding cut quality and ease of tissue separation was found between two ranges.

ID	Sphere/lenticule thickness	Flap energy/lenticule energy	Track distance/spot distance (μm)
7	−5 D/96 μm	Index 22	3.5/3.5
8	−10 D/166 μm	Index 22	3.5/3.5
15	−5 D/96 μm	Index 40	5.0/5.0
16	−10 D/166 μm	Index 40	5.0/5.0

Next we reduced the energy with the recommended spot and tracking distance from index 28 to index 24. The result was a slightly better UDVA on the first day after treatment, but without any significance.

Furthermore we enlarged the recommended spot and tracking distance using identical energy level (index 24/26) from 3.0 to 3.8 μ. The result was a significant better UDVA on the first day postoperatively.

From this we concluded that a decrease of energy per area might be the key for optimized settings. In a next step we decreased the energy level per area from 4.1 μ/index 36 to 4.5 μ/index 36.

Our findings:

- Easier lenticule extraction by increasing spot and tracking distance
- No critical low energy level, which might lead to uncontrolled tissue separation
- Better adjustment possible due to higher energy level
- Significant better results of UDVA (1 day post-op)
- Shorter treatment time with reduced risk of suction loss

The results are summarized and displayed in Figs. 11.1, 11.2, and 11.3.

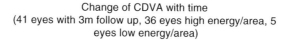

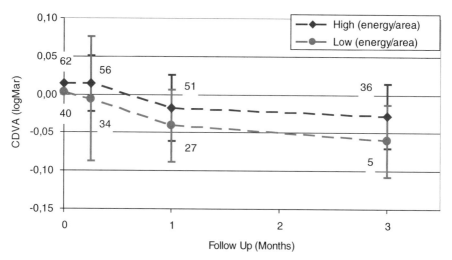

Fig. 11.1 A direct comparison of CDVA between the two different energy per area groups

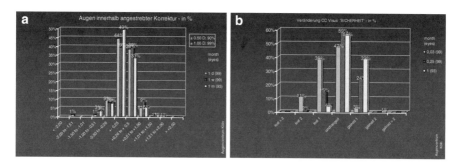

Fig. 11.2 (**a**) (*Left hand side*) shows the predictability of refractive change and (**b**) shows safety (CDVA; *right side*) at 1st day, 1st week, and 1st month before adjustment of the laser settings

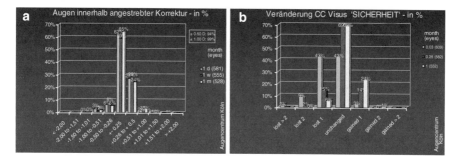

Fig. 11.3 (**a**) (*Left hand side*) shows the predictability of refractive change and (**b**) shows the safety (CDVA; *right hand side*) at 1st day, 1st week, and 1st month after adjustment of the laser settings. Higher accuracy and slightly better safety at all early follow up checks

Conclusion

As a result of our tests we can summarize that the application of a 4.5 μ spot and tracking distance with an energy level of 180 nJ per spot results in an optimized low energy density for a minimized tissue distortion and an easy lenticule extraction with the current 500 kHz VisuMax laser. Meanwhile these adjusted settings are implemented in the VisuMax femtosecond laser by Carl Zeiss Meditec.

Moreover, in our daily clinical practice patients take effective advantages of these new settings:

- Shorter treatment time (up to 30 %, less risk of suction loss)
- Faster visual recovery (esp. UDVA 1st day post-op)
- More precise refraction on the first day postoperatively
- Less tissue affection direct postoperatively (edema, stromal disorders)

Reference

1. Shah R, Shah S (2011) Effect of scanning patterns on the results of femtosecond laser lenticule extraction refractive surgery. J Cataract Refract Surg 37:1636–1647

Advantages and Disadvantages of Different Cap Thicknesses

12

Jose L. Güell[$], Paula Verdaguer[$], Honorio Pallás, Daniel Elies, Oscar Gris, and Felicidad Manero

Contents

12.1 Introduction

The small incision lenticule extraction (SMILE) procedure is an all-in-one technology for correcting refractive errors that has become available for intrastromal lenticule cutting and subsequent lenticule extraction. SMILE technology has

[$]Author contributed equally with all other contributors.

Electronic supplementary material The online version of this chapter (doi:10.1007/978-3-319-18530-9_12) contains supplementary material, which is available to authorized users.

J.L. Güell, MD, PhD • P. Verdaguer, MD (✉) • D. Elies, MD • O. Gris, MD, PhD
Department of Ophthalmology, Cornea and Refractive Surgery Unit,
Instituto de Microcirugia Ocular (IMO), c/Josep Maria Lladó 3, 08035 Barcelona, Spain

"Universitat Autònoma de Barcelona" (UAB), Barcelona, Spain
e-mail: guell@imo.es; paulaverdaguer@gmail.com

H. Pallás • F. Manero, MD
Department of Ophthalmology, Cornea and Refractive Surgery Unit,
Instituto de Microcirugia Ocular (IMO), c/Josep Maria Lladó 3, 08035 Barcelona, Spain

© Springer International Publishing Switzerland 2015
W. Sekundo (ed.), *Small Incision Lenticule Extraction (SMILE):
Principles, Techniques, Complication Management, and Future Concepts*,
DOI 10.1007/978-3-319-18530-9_12

exhibited excellent efficacy, safety, and predictability for the correction of myopia and astigmatism [1, 2].

We started using the SMILE technique in 2011 with progressively better visual and refractive results. Taking into account the theoretically lower impact on corneal biomechanics with deeper cuts and with the concept in mind of a secondary more superficial re-SMILE, we decided to study the refractive and visual results of deeper lenticule depths. The procedure was performed using four different lenticule depths in a prospective, non-randomized way (130, 140, 150, and 160 μm).

12.2   Surgical Procedure

A standard SMILE surgery sequence as described in Chaps. 5 and 6 was carried out. At the conclusion of the laser scan an opening incision of 30° length (approx. 2 mm) was created at the 10.30-o'clock position for lenticule extraction. The shape of the lenticule generated was designed to correct the refractive error. The femtosecond laser parameters were adjusted for 130, 140, 150, or 160 μm cap thickness, 7.5 mm diameter of anterior lenticule surface, 6.5 mm diameter of posterior lenticule surface, and at the VisuMax energy level of 26 and spot/track distance of 3 μm for both the lenticule and cap cuts. We increased the spherical equivalent of the correction by 3 % for every 10 μm of higher depth in relation to the 130 μm cap. After completion of the laser sequence, a blunt spatula (G-33954 Güell Femto Double-Ended instrument, Geuder GmbH, Germany) was inserted through the small incision over the roof of the refractive lenticule dissecting this plane, followed by the bottom of the lenticule. The lenticule was subsequently grasped and removed with micro forceps. After removal of the lenticule, the stromal pocket was flushed with BSS using a Güell flap hydrodissection cannula 25G (AE-7288) (Video 12.1).

12.3   Postoperative Treatment

Standard postoperative treatment was tobramycin antibiotic and dexamethasone steroid eye drops (Tobradex™, Alcon) tid for a week and then slowly tapered off over a 4-week period, plus preservative-free artificial tears five times a day for almost a month.

12.4   Statistical Analysis

Microsoft Excel (Microsoft; Redmond, Washington, USA) was used for data collection and for performing descriptive statistics. Continuous variables were described with mean and standard deviation (SD).

The results were analyzed using SPSS software version 17.0 (SPSS Inc., Chicago, Illinois, USA). Comparison between preoperative and postoperative data was performed using Wilcoxon signed-rank tests for nonparametric data. The tests were performed before surgery, at 4 weeks (1 month), 3 months, 6 months, and at 1 year after the surgery. A p-value lower than 0.05 was considered to be statistically significant.

12.5   Results

Ninety-four eyes of 47 patients with myopia with and without myopic astigmatism were recruited for this study. The number of eyes in the four different lenticule-depth groups were 130 μm ($n=44$), 140 μm ($n=14$), 150 μm ($n=12$), and 160 μm ($n=24$). Mean preoperative logMAR uncorrected visual acuity (UCVA) was 1.21 (SD 0.35). Mean postoperative logMAR UCVA was 0.15 (SD 0.20) at 1 month, 0.08 (SD 0.12) at 3 months, 0.07 (SD 0.12) at 6 months, and 0.07 (SD 0.12) at 1 year. There were no statistically significant differences in the UCVA variables between the four groups ($p<0.05$).

Mean preoperative spherical equivalent (SE) was −4.89 (SD 1.48). Mean postoperative SE was −0.26 (SD 0.42) at 1 month, −0.24 (SD 0.39) at 3 months, 0.09 (SD 0.62) at 6 months, and 0.07 (SD 0.57) at 1 year. There were no statistically significant differences in the SE variable between the four groups ($p<0.05$).

Mean preoperative cylinder (CYL) was −0.63 (SD 0.54). Mean postoperative CYL was −0.28 (SD 0.47) at 1 month, −0.21 (SD 0.41) at 3 months, −0.33 (SD 0.42) at 6 months, and −0.16 (SD 0.34) at 1 year. There were no significant statistical differences in CYL when the different groups were compared for the same periods of time ($p<0.05$).

We did not observe statistically significant differences using the SMILE technique at four different lenticule depths in a random manner (130, 140, 150, and 160 μm) in visual acuity or refractive outcomes (Figs. 12.1, 12.2, and 12.3) with a minimum follow-up time of 1 year.

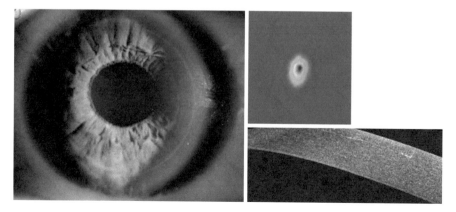

Fig. 12.1 Anterior segment photography of an eye 3 months post 130 μm SMILE procedure. Anterior segment optical coherence tomography and Optical Quality Analysis System (OQAS) (Visometrics SL, Terrassa, Barcelona) of the same eye

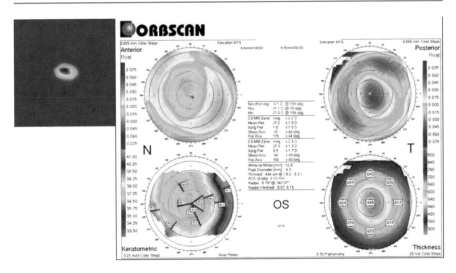

Fig. 12.2 Orbscan (Orbtek Inc./Bausch & Lomb, Tampa, FL, USA) corneal topography and OQAS of one left eye 3 months post 140 μm SMILE procedure

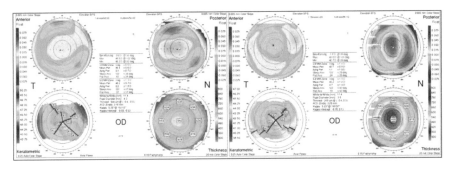

Fig. 12.3 Orbscan (Orbtek Inc./Bausch & Lomb, Tampa, FL, USA) corneal topography of one right eye pre- and 3 months post 160 μm procedure

In some cases, we had more difficulties in dissecting the stroma as deeper was the cut in some cases but not in all of them. That is why we cannot make a significant difference also in this point.

No complications were observed during the surgery and the immediate postoperative period.

12.6   Discussion

SMILE has good refractive outcomes and other benefits such as reduction in scatter. This procedure induces fewer higher-order aberrations and exerts a minimal negative impact on the quality of the retinal image leading to good vision [3–6].

Moreover, it is less invasive and there is a reduction in postoperative irritation, less loss of corneal sensitivity, less inflammation, and less impact on tear production, because the short incision cuts fewer corneal nerves (see Chaps. 2 and 3). In addition, tissue extraction is more precise and repeatable regardless of the treatment prescription. As no flap is created, there is a potential better postoperative biomechanical stability and a lesser risk of secondary corneal ectasia, due to the preservation of the anterior corneal stromal layer, which in turn preserves corneal resistance (see Chap. 13) [7–9].

Dry eye is a common complaint among patients who have undergone refractive surgery, including laser in situ keratomileusis (LASIK), photorefractive keratectomy, and femtosecond LASIK whereby and the incidence of dry eye varies among these different patients [7–11]. It has been reported that patients who develop dry eye after refractive surgery also have elevated risks of developing subsequent refractive regression and ocular surface damage. In addition, refractive surgery procedures also interrupt the normal organization and regeneration of the corneal nerves, which in turn lead to a prolonged reduction in corneal sensation (see Chap. 3).

A recent study added an important issue that surgery could result in dry eye symptoms, tear film instability, and decreased corneal sensitivity. Furthermore, SMILE has superiority over Femto-LASIK in lower risk of postoperative corneal fluorescein staining and less reduction of corneal sensation [12].

As no flap is created with the SMILE technique, there is theoretically a higher postoperative biomechanical stability and a lower risk of secondary corneal ectasia due to the anatomical preservation of the anterior corneal stromal layer. The treatment is carried out under Bowman's layer, which creates greater corneal resistance. Several authors argue that – from the biomechanical point of view – in a cornea operated on by LASIK surgery, the useful corneal thickness is that of the residual stromal bed, as the flap thickness is not important when it comes to maintaining the corneal structure: corneal weakening is greater when the residual stromal thickness is thinner (the recommended residual stromal thickness is 250–300 µm) [12–14]. With the SMILE technique, this concept changes: because of the preservation of Bowman's layer, a greater lenticule depth (= a thicker cap) shell go along with more corneal resistance [13, 14].

Conversely, it is possible that being deeper leads to a lower precision of the femtosecond laser cut diminishing the refractive predictability of the procedure. To overcome this possible energy loss and following discussions with the company, we decided to increase 3 % of the spherical equivalent correction for every 10 µm of higher depth in relation to the 130 µm cap. That regularly meant that for all of our 160 µm depth SMILE we were correcting 10 % higher.

Despite different cap thicknesses, there were no additional complications either in regard to the surgical technique or any parameters of visual quality or refraction, safety, and predictability between the four lenticule depth groups (130, 140, 150, and 160µm) at the different follow-ups.

Another aim of the study was to find out if we could perform a second more superficial SMILE procedure in case of a possible retreatment. Current retreatment techniques are summarized in Chap. 10. Conceptually, after a SMILE procedure at 160 µm depth, one could repeat SMILE at 130 µm. This concept has already been tested by our group in two cases of primary SMILE at 160 μm and retreatment with re-SMILE at 130 μm achieving good refractive and visual results. As a matter of case these two cases showed a residual refraction of >−1 D (which in our opinion is the minimum refraction needed to perform a SMILE treatment), because we initially aimed for monovision, but the patients complained of discomfort in binocular vision (submitted for publication as case report).

Our study also confirmed the assumption that in order to obtain the same refractive results at 160 μm as compared to 130 μm, it was necessary to apply an additional 10 % of correction without changes in laser energy settings.

In summary, the present study shows no differences in visual acuity, refractive outcomes, and optical visual quality using the four different cap thicknesses. Setting a primary SMILE procedure at 160μm might lead to a better corneal stability and leave enough anterior stroma for a secondary SMILE retreatment at 130 μm or thinner.

Further comparative studies are required to support these conclusions in order to decide the ideal depth for primary and secondary SMILE procedures.

References

1. Vestergaard A, Ivarsen A, Asp S, Hjortdal J (2013) Femtosecond (FS) laser vision correction procedure for moderate to high myopia: a prospective study of ReLExflex and comparison with a retrospective study of FS-laser in situ keratomileusis. Acta Ophthalmol 91(4):355–362
2. Verdaguer P, El-Husseiny MA, Elies D, Gris O, Manero F, Biarnés M, Güell JL (2013) Small incision lenticule extraction (SMILE) procedure for the correction of myopia and myopic astigmatism. J Emmetropia 4:191–196
3. Sekundo W, Kunert KS, Blum M (2011) Small incision corneal refractive surgery using the small incision lenticule extraction (SMILE) procedure for the correction of myopia and myopic astigmatism: results of a 6 month prospective study. Br J Ophthalmol 95(3):335–339
4. Vestergaard A, Ivarsen A, Asp S, Hjortdal J (2012) ReLEx smile for moderate to high myopia: a prospective study of predictability, safety and patient satisfaction. J Cataract Refract Surg 38(11):2003–2010
5. Hjortdal J, Vestergaard AH, Ivarsen A, Ragunathan S, Asp S (2012) Predictors for the outcome of small incision lenticule extraction for myopia. Journal of Refractive Surgery 28(12): 865–871
6. Miao H, He L, Shen Y, Li M, Yu Y, Zhou X (2014) Optical quality and intraocular scattering after femtosecond laser small incision lenticule extraction. J Refract Surg 30(5):296–302
7. Wu D, Wang Y, Zhang L, Wei S, Tang X (2014) Corneal biomechanical effects: small-incision lenticule extraction versus femtosecond laser-assisted laser in situ keratomileusis. J Cataract Refract Surg 40(6):954–962
8. Kamiya K, Shimizu K, Igarashi A, Kobashi H (2014) Visual and refractive outcomes of femtosecond lenticule extraction and small-incision lenticule extraction for myopia. Am J Ophthalmol 157(1):128–134
9. Gatinel D, Chaabouni S, Adam PA, Munck J, Puech M, Hoang-Xuan T (2007) Corneal Hysteresis, resistance factor, topography, and pachymetry after corneal lamellar flap. J Refract Surg 23:76–84
10. Chang DH, Stulting RD (2005) Change in intraocular pressure measurements after LASIK the effect of the refractive correction and the lamellar flap. Ophthalmology 112:1009–1016
11. Ivarsen A, Asp S, Hjortdal J (2014) Safety and complications of more than 1500 small-incision lenticule extraction procedures. Ophthalmology 121(4):822–828

12. Li M, Zhao J, Shen Y, Li T, He L, Xu H, Yu Y, Zhou X (2013) Comparison of dry eye and corneal sensitivity between small incision lenticule extraction and femtosecond LASIK for myopia. PLoS One 8(10):e77797
13. Sekundo W, Gertnere J, Bertelmann T, Solomatin I (2014) One-year refractive results, contrast sensitivity, high-order aberrations and complications after myopic small-incision lenticule extraction (ReLEx SMILE). Graefes Arch Clin Exp Ophthalmol 252(5):837–843
14. Kamiya K, Shimizu K, Igarashi A, Kobashi H, Sato N, Ishii R (2014) Intraindividual comparison of changes in corneal biomechanical parameters after femtosecond lenticule extraction and small-incision lenticule extraction. J Cataract Refract Surg 40(6):963–970

The Key Characteristics of Corneal Refractive Surgery: Biomechanics, Spherical Aberration, and Corneal Sensitivity After SMILE

13

Dan Z. Reinstein, Timothy J. Archer, and Marine Gobbe

Contents

Financial Disclosure Dr Reinstein is a consultant for Carl Zeiss Meditec (Jena, Germany) and has a proprietary interest in the Artemis technology (ArcScan Inc., Morrison, Colorado) and is an author of patents related to VHF digital ultrasound administered by the Cornell Center for Technology Enterprise and Commercialization (CCTEC), Ithaca, New York. The remaining authors have no proprietary or financial interest in the materials presented herein.

D.Z. Reinstein, MD, MA(Cantab), FRCOphth (✉)
Refractive Surgery, London Vision Clinic, 138 Harley Street, London, UK

Department of Ophthalmology, Columbia University Medical Center, New York, NY, USA

Department of d'Ophthalmologie, Centre Hospitalier National d'Ophtalmologie, Paris, France
e-mail: dzr@londonvisionclinic.com

T.J. Archer, MA(Oxon), DipCompSci(Cantab) • M. Gobbe, MSTOptom, PhD
Refractive Surgery, London Vision Clinic, 138 Harley Street, London, UK
e-mail: tim@londonvisionclinic.com; marine@londonvisionclinic.com

© Springer International Publishing Switzerland 2015
W. Sekundo (ed.), *Small Incision Lenticule Extraction (SMILE):*
Principles, Techniques, Complication Management, and Future Concepts,
DOI 10.1007/978-3-319-18530-9_13

13.1 Potential Biomechanical Advantages of SMILE

One of the potential benefits of the SMILE procedure is increased biomechanical stability due to the absence of a flap. There are two main reasons for this:

1. Vertical cuts (e.g., flap side cut) have more biomechanical impact than horizontal cuts.
2. Anterior stromal lamellae are stronger than posterior stromal lamellae.

13.1.1 Vertical Cuts Have More Biomechanical Impact than Horizontal Cuts

In 2000, we published the first paper showing in vivo that the peripheral stroma actually thickens after LASIK, as shown in Fig. 13.1 [1]. This biomechanical change seems to be a true cause for the majority of spherical aberration induction (probably about 85 %) rather than the more commonly discussed reasons of laser fluence projection and reflection errors in the periphery due to the curvature of the cornea. This finding agreed with the results reported by Dupps and Roberts [2, 3] of peripheral stromal thickening outside the treatment zone after phototherapeutic keratectomy (PTK) in ex vivo human donor globes.

Dupps and Roberts had also proposed a model to explain this finding [3, 4]. Briefly, the cornea is made of layers of collagen lamellae running from limbus to limbus oriented at precise angles with respect to adjacent lamellae, contributing to corneal transparency and strength. Stromal collagen lamellae are surrounded by several proteoglycans responsible for proper spacing of collagen and stromal hydration. The creation of a flap and stromal tissue ablation severs the anterior corneal

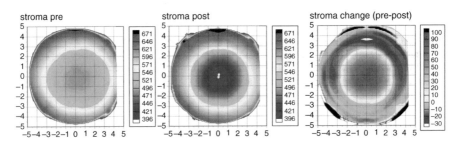

Fig. 13.1 Artemis® very high-frequency digital ultrasound (ArcScan Inc.) stromal thickness maps before (*left*) and 3 months after (*middle*) LASIK for −9.00 D myopia using the MEL80 excimer laser (Carl Zeiss Meditec) with a 6 mm optical zone. The color scales are thickness in µm and a Cartesian grid is superimposed at 1 mm intervals for the 10 mm diameter. Scans were centered on the corneal vertex. The difference map (*right*) shows the change in stromal thickness (*red/orange* represents stromal thinning, *blue/green* represents stromal thickening) demonstrating the tissue removed by the ablation centrally with less tissue removal radially as expected for a myopic ablation. However, outside the 6 mm optical zone, the stroma was actually thicker after LASIK

Table 13.1 Percentage increase in central corneal strain (to an intraocular pressure change from 15 to 15.5 mmHg) after the creation of a LASIK flap, a side cut, or delamination at both 90 and 160 μm

	90 μm	160 μm
LASIK flap	9 %	32 %
Side cut only	9 %	33 %
Delamination only	5 %	5 %

Data obtained from Knox Cartwright et al. [5]

lamellae, which means that the peripheral anterior lamellae are no longer under tension and therefore relax and spread out resulting in stromal thickening. The consequence of this expansion of peripheral anterior lamellae is to exert a pulling force on the posterior lamellae, which causes central flattening. However, the posterior lamellae also have to contend with an unchanged IOP, which can result in some forward bowing of the cornea.

Recently, Knox Cartwright et al. [5] reported a study on human cadaver eyes in organ culture that compared the corneal strain produced by a LASIK flap, a side cut only, and a delamination cut only, with each incision type performed at both 90 and 160 μm. Table 13.1 summarizes the results, which found that the increase in strain was equivalent between a LASIK flap and a side cut alone at both depths with a significantly greater increase for the 160 μm depth. In contrast, the increase in strain after a delamination cut only (i.e., no vertical side cut) was lower than after a LASIK flap or side cut only. Also, the strain did not increase when a delamination cut only was performed at the greater 160 μm depth. A similar result has also been found in a study by Medeiros et al. [6] who showed in pig eyes that there was significantly greater biomechanical changes following the creation of a thick flap of 300 μm compared to a thin flap of 100 μm.

Applying this finding to SMILE, since no anterior corneal side cut is created, there will be slightly less increase in corneal strain in SMILE compared to thin flap LASIK and a significant difference in corneal strain compared to LASIK with a thicker flap.

13.1.2 Anterior Stromal Lamellae Are Stronger than Posterior Stromal Lamellae

Randleman et al. [7] demonstrated that the cohesive tensile strength (i.e., how strongly the stromal lamellae are held together) of the stroma decreases from anterior to posterior within the central corneal region (Fig. 13.2). In an experiment in which the cohesive tensile strength was measured for strips of stromal lamellae cut from different depths within donor corneoscleral buttons, a strong negative correlation was found between stromal depth and cohesive tensile strength. The anterior 40 % of the central corneal stroma was found to be the strongest region of the cornea, whereas the posterior 60 % of the stroma was at least 50 % weaker. A number of other authors have reached this conclusion by other indirect means [8–13].

Fig. 13.2 Scatter plots of the percentage of maximum cohesive tensile strength against the percentage of residual stromal depth using data from the study by Randleman et al. [7]. Regression analysis found that a fourth-order polynomial provided the closest fit to the data and the R^2 of 0.93 demonstrated the high correlation achieved. The fourth-order polynomial regression equation was integrated to calculate the area under the curve for the relevant stromal depths after photorefractive keratectomy (*PRK*), LASIK, and small incision lenticule extraction (*SMILE*) as demonstrated by the green shaded regions. The *red areas* represent the tissue removed (excimer laser ablation/lenticule extraction) and the purple area in LASIK represents the LASIK flap (Reprinted with permission from Reinstein et al. [24])

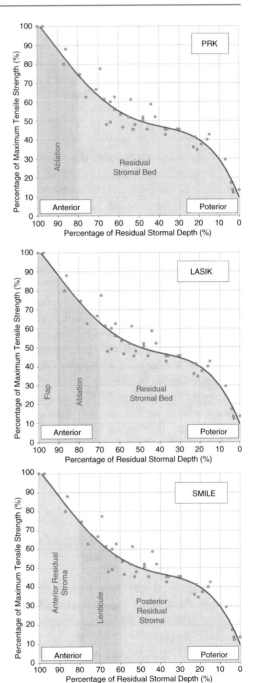

Fig. 13.3 Tangential tensile strength (longitudinal modulus of elasticity) measured by Brillouin microscopy at different depths in a (bovine) cornea including the epithelium (I), anterior stroma (II), posterior stroma (III), and the innermost region near the endothelium (IV) (Reprinted with permission from Scarcelli et al. [15])

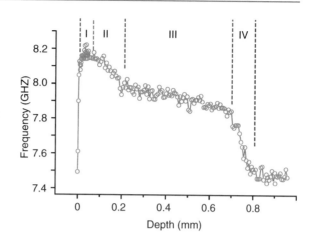

In addition to cohesive tensile strength, tangential tensile strength (i.e., stiffness along the stromal lamellae) and shear strength (i.e., resistance to torsional forces) have both been found to vary with depth in the stroma. Kohlhaas et al. [14] and Scarcelli et al. [15] found that the tangential tensile strength was greater for anterior stroma than posterior stroma, each using different methodology. Petsche et al. [16] found a similar result for transverse shear strength to decrease with stromal depth. The same group have used nonlinear optical high-resolution macroscopy to image the three-dimensional distribution of transverse collagen fibers and have shown that the nonlinearity of tensile strength through the stroma is caused by the greater interconnectivity of the collagen fibers in the anterior stroma compared with the posterior stroma where the collagen fibers lie in parallel to each other [17].

An interesting finding of these studies is the nonlinear nature of the change in tensile strength through the stroma. The cohesive tensile strength appears to decrease rapidly for the anterior-most 30 % [7]. There is then a region between 70 and 20 % depth where the cohesive tensile strength decreases slowly, but then drops off sharply again for the posterior-most 20 %. This nonlinearity may be associated with the known different collagen organizational layers within the stroma [10, 18, 19]. Of note is the remarkable similarity of this curve to that reported for tangential tensile strength by Scarcelli et al. [15] (Fig. 13.3), which demonstrates the strong correlation between corneal biomechanical properties with stromal depth. This finding also agrees with studies that have found other depth-dependent properties of the corneal stroma such as decreasing refractive index [20], greater UV-B absorption in the anterior stroma [21], and varying excimer laser ablation rates [22, 23].

13.1.3 Paradigm Shift in Residual Stromal Thickness Calculation

We are accustomed to calculating the residual stromal thickness in LASIK as the amount of stromal tissue left under the flap, so the first instinct is to apply this rule to SMILE. However, the actual residual stromal thickness in SMILE should be calculated as the stromal thickness below the posterior lenticule interface *plus* the stromal thickness between the anterior lenticule interface and Bowman's layer since the anterior stromal lamellae have not been cut, except in the location of the small incision. So the first change is that we need to consider the total uncut stromal thickness in SMILE as opposed to the LASIK residual stromal bed thickness.

But given that SMILE effectively leaves anterior corneal stroma intact, while the keratomileusis takes place in the deeper and therefore weaker portion of the cornea (as described above), it is reasonable to assume that for any given refractive correction, SMILE will leave the cornea with greater tensile strength than either LASIK or PRK. To take this into account, we need to start thinking more in terms of tensile strength rather than simply in terms of residual stromal thickness. For example, a rough adjustment would be to say that anterior stroma is approximately 50 % stronger than posterior stroma, so a further 50 % of the untouched anterior stromal thickness in SMILE can be added to get an adjusted total uncut stromal thickness value that can be compared to a LASIK residual stromal bed thickness. In reality, we can go further than this by basing the calculation on the real stromal tensile strength data.

13.1.4 Biomechanics Model: Comparing SMILE to PRK and LASIK

We recently developed a mathematical model based directly on the Randleman [7] depth-dependent tensile strength data to calculate the postoperative tensile strength and compare this between PRK, LASIK, and SMILE [24]. Given the similarity between different studies measuring the different types of tensile strength as described above, we made the assumption that cohesive tensile strength is representative of the overall corneal biomechanics. We now suggest that this total tensile strength value should replace residual stromal thickness as the limiting factor for corneal refractive surgery.

To derive the model, first we performed nonlinear regression analysis on the Randleman [7] data and found that a fourth-order curve maximized the fit to the data with an R^2 of 0.930 demonstrating the very high correlation achieved by a nonlinear fit. The total tensile strength of the untreated cornea was then calculated as the area under the regression line by integration (see Fig. 13.2). The total tensile strength of the cornea after LASIK was derived by calculating the area under the regression line for all depths below the residual stromal bed thickness (assuming the flap does not contribute to the tensile strength of the postoperative cornea [25]). This value was divided by the total tensile strength of the untreated cornea to represent the relative postoperative total tensile strength (PTTS) as a percentage. Similarly, the total tensile strength of the cornea after PRK was derived by calculating the area under the regression line for all depths below the stromal thickness after ablation. Finally, the total tensile strength of the cornea after SMILE was calculated as the area under the regression line for all depths below the lower lenticule interface added to the area under the regression line for all depths above the upper lenticule interface or within the stromal cap.

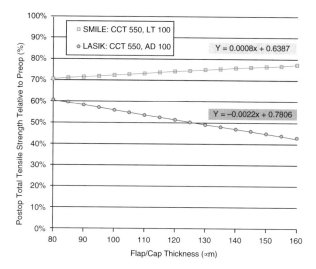

Fig. 13.4 Scatter plot of the relative total tensile strength after LASIK (*purple*) and small incision lenticule extraction (SMILE) (*green*) plotted against a range of flap/cap thicknesses for a fixed central corneal thickness of 550 μm and ablation depth/lenticule thickness of 100 μm (approximately −7.75 D). In LASIK, the postoperative relative total tensile strength decreased for greater flap thickness by 0.22 %/μm. In SMILE, the postoperative relative total tensile strength increased for greater cap thickness by 0.08 %/μm (Reprinted with permission from Reinstein et al. [24])

The model was then applied to a variety of different scenarios and a number of conclusions could be drawn from the analyses:

1. As would be expected, the postoperative tensile strength was greater after SMILE than after LASIK – because the anterior stroma is left intact, SMILE will (by definition) leave the cornea with greater tensile strength than LASIK for any given refractive correction.
2. The postoperative tensile strength was greater after SMILE than after PRK – in SMILE, the refractive stromal tissue removal takes place in deeper and relatively weaker stroma, leaving the stronger anterior stroma intact, meaning that for any given refractive correction, SMILE will leave the cornea with greater tensile strength than PRK.
3. The postoperative tensile strength increased for SMILE with increasing cap thickness (Fig. 13.4) – if SMILE is performed deeper in the cornea, more of the stronger anterior stroma will remain and hence the postoperative tensile strength will be greater; this is in contrast to LASIK, where a thicker flap results in lower postoperative tensile strength given the minimal contribution of the flap to corneal biomechanics after healing.
4. The postoperative tensile strength decreased for thinner corneas, but the difference between procedures also increased for thinner corneas (Fig. 13.5) – for example, in LASIK, flap stroma plus ablation within the stronger anterior stroma would comprise a greater percentage loss of total tensile strength than lenticular

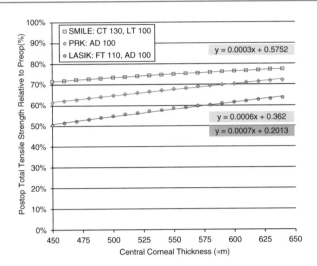

Fig. 13.5 Scatter plot comparing total tensile strength for a fixed ablation with varying corneal thicknesses after LASIK (*purple*), photorefractive keratectomy (PRK) (*blue*), and small incision lenticule extraction (SMILE) (*green*) against a range of central corneal thickness for a fixed ablation depth/lenticule thickness of 100 μm (approximately −7.75 D), a LASIK flap thickness of 110 μm, and a SMILE cap thickness of 130 μm. The postoperative relative total tensile strength was greatest after SMILE, followed by PRK, and was lowest after LASIK (Reprinted with permission from Reinstein et al. [24])

removal from relatively weaker stromal tissue deeper within the stroma while leaving stronger anterior stroma uncut.

These results can be quantified in the example scenario represented in Fig. 13.6 which shows the relative total tensile strength after LASIK (purple), photorefractive keratectomy (PRK) (blue), and small incision lenticule extraction (SMILE) (green) plotted against a range of ablation depths for a fixed central corneal thickness of 550 μm, a LASIK flap thickness of 110 μm, and a SMILE cap thickness of 130 μm. The *orange lines* indicate that the postoperative relative total tensile strength reached 60 % for an ablation depth of 73 μm in LASIK (approximately −5.75 diopters [D]), 132 μm in PRK (approximately −10.00 D), and 175 μm in SMILE (approximately −13.50 D), translating to a 7.75 D difference between LASIK and SMILE for a cornea of the same postoperative relative total tensile strength. The red lines indicate that the postoperative relative total tensile strength after a 100 μm tissue removal would be 54 % in LASIK, 68 % in PRK, and 75 % in SMILE.

In this model, there are some factors that have not been considered. First, this model only considers the central point on the cornea. A full model of the cornea, for example, by finite element analysis, that can take into account the stromal thickness progression and the volume of the ablation profile would be a significant improvement but is likely to provide the same data qualitatively, albeit perhaps more accurately in terms of absolute tensile strength changes. Indeed, one study has used finite element modeling to compare the stress distribution after SMILE and LASIK and found that there was a greater increase in the stress in the residual stromal bed in the LASIK model than in the SMILE model [27].

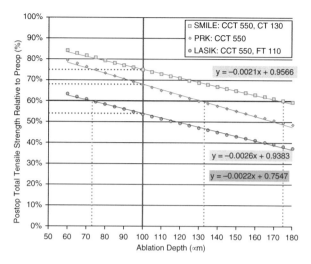

Fig. 13.6 This graph shows the relative total tensile strength after LASIK (*purple*), photorefractive keratectomy (PRK) (*blue*), and small incision lenticule extraction (SMILE) (*green*) plotted against a range of ablation depths for a fixed central corneal thickness of 550 μm, a LASIK flap thickness of 110 μm, and a SMILE cap thickness of 130 μm. The *orange lines* indicate that the postoperative relative total tensile strength reached 60 % for an ablation depth of 73 μm in LASIK (approximately −5.75 diopters [D]), 132 μm in PRK (approximately −10.00 D), and 175 μm in SMILE (approximately −13.50 D), translating to a 7.75 D difference between LASIK and SMILE for a cornea of the same postoperative relative total tensile strength. The red lines indicate that the postoperative relative total tensile strength after a 100 μm tissue removal would be 54 % in LASIK, 68 % in PRK, and 75 % in SMILE (Reprinted with permission from Reinstein et al. [24])

In the model, we have made the assumption that the stromal lamellae in the LASIK flap do not contribute to the total tensile strength of the cornea at all, an assumption that is supported by published studies demonstrating negligible contribution. Schmack et al. [25] found that the mean tensile strength of the central and paracentral LASIK wounds was only 2.4 % that measured in the control eyes. As described earlier, Knox Cartwright et al. [5] experimentally demonstrated a LASIK flap depth-dependent increase in corneal strain, reporting an increase in strain of 9 % for a 110 μm flap and 33 % for a 160 μm flap. This result is predicted by our current model which showed that the remaining relative total tensile strength would be less for thicker flaps, as would be expected.

Another factor not considered is that Bowman's layer remains intact after SMILE, which is not true in either LASIK or PRK. Bowman's layer has been shown to have very different biomechanical properties to stromal tissue as demonstrated by Seiler et al. [26] who showed that removing Bowman's layer with an excimer laser reduced Young's modulus by 4.75 %. Leaving Bowman's layer intact may further increase the corneal biomechanical stability after SMILE compared with LASIK and PRK. Finally, the present model in addition does not consider the effect of the tunnel incision on tensile strength changes which although small will not be zero.

In summary, considering the safety of subtractive corneal refractive surgical procedures in terms of tensile strength represents a paradigm shift away from classical residual stromal thickness limits. The residual thickness-based safety of corneal laser refractive surgery should be thought of at least in terms of total residual uncut stroma. Ideally, a parameter such as total tensile strength, which takes the nonlinearity of the strength of the stroma into account, seems more appropriate. For example, the residual stromal bed thickness under the interface in SMILE could easily be less than 250 μm due to the additional strength provided by the untouched stromal lamellae in the cap, as long as the total remaining corneal tensile strength is comparable to that of the post-LASIK 250 μm residual stromal bed thickness standard. In this new case of using remaining total tensile strength, the minimum would evidently be defined as the total tensile strength remaining after LASIK with a residual stromal bed thickness of 250 μm.

13.2   Evidence for Biomechanical Advantages of SMILE

As described earlier, spherical aberration induction is largely due to peripheral stromal expansion outside the ablation zone. Peripheral stromal expansion is caused by the relaxation of severed stromal collagen lamellae, so it would be expected to find less stromal expansion after SMILE as fewer lamellae are cut, and hence, it would be expected for less spherical aberration to be induced.

In a recent study [33], we compared the induction of spherical aberration between SMILE, where the refractive lenticule is only minimally aspheric, and LASIK using the MEL80 with the Laser Blended Vision module [29], which uses a nonlinear aspherically optimized ablation profile. The LASIK group was matched by refraction to within ±0.25 D and all eyes were treated with a 6 mm optical zone in both groups. Corneal spherical aberration (Atlas, Carl Zeiss Meditec) was analyzed for a 6 mm diameter and no difference was found between the two groups. Therefore, SMILE though minimally aspheric produced similar spherical aberration induction to the highly aspherically optimized myopic Laser Blended Vision profile. This indicates that the femtosecond flapless procedure leads to less induction of spherical aberration than expected for a non-aspheric conventional excimer myopic profile. These results are similar to other published studies: two studies have shown that there are less aberrations induced by SMILE than LASIK [30, 31], and one study showed that induction of aberrations was similar [32].

Following this study, we also investigated how the induction of spherical aberration after SMILE changed for optical zones of 6, 6.5, and 7 mm. The induced spherical aberration decreased as expected for larger SMILE optical zones; the regression line slope was 0.081 for 6 mm, 0.059 for 6.5 mm, and 0.030 for 7 mm (Fig. 13.7).

But another factor to be considered is the ablation depth. Due to the aspheric optimization of the Laser Blended Vision ablation profiles, the ablation depth is greater than the SMILE lenticule thickness for the same optical zone; a 6 mm Laser Blended Vision ablation is equivalent to a 6.25 mm SMILE lenticule in terms of stromal tissue removal. Therefore, since we know that spherical aberration induction decreases for larger optical zones, spherical aberration induction after SMILE is significantly less than LASIK for an equivalent stromal tissue removal.

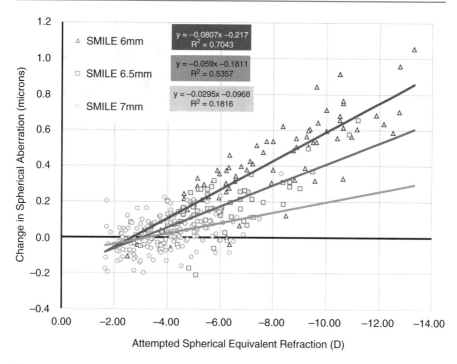

Fig. 13.7 Scatter plot showing the change in spherical aberration (OSA notation) plotted against the spherical equivalent refraction treated by SMILE in a 6, 6.5, and 7 mm optical zone

Finally, we need to also consider the biomechanical difference between the two procedures as described earlier. According to our model, the difference in tensile strength is enough that the cornea is still significantly stronger after SMILE than LASIK even when a much larger optical zone is used in SMILE (i.e., greater tissue removal). Further increasing the optical zone enables less spherical aberration induction, and therefore, better optical quality can be achieved while still leaving the cornea stronger.

To demonstrate this, we retrospectively applied the model to our initial SMILE case series ($n=96$) and compared the postoperative total tensile strength to a control group of LASIK eyes matched for refraction (±0.25 D) and pachymetry (±20 μm) [33]. Optical zone was not part of the matching criteria, so that the populations represented routine clinical use of the two procedures. Mean optical zone was 6.70 ± 0.39 mm (range 5.90–7.00 mm) for the SMILE group and 6.08 ± 0.22 mm (range 5.75–7.00 mm) for the LASIK group. Mean ablation depth was 107 ± 19 μm (range 72–149 μm) for the SMILE group and 87 ± 25 μm (range 25–134 μm) for the LASIK group. Mean SMILE cap thickness was 130 μm (range 120–140 μm). Mean LASIK flap thickness was 96 μm (range 80–120 μm). Mean spherical equivalent refraction was -4.83 ± 1.59 D (range up to -8.00 D) for both groups. Mean central corneal pachymetry was 539 ± 30 μm (range 468–591 μm) for the SMILE group and 545 ± 36 μm (range 469–626 μm) for the LASIK group.

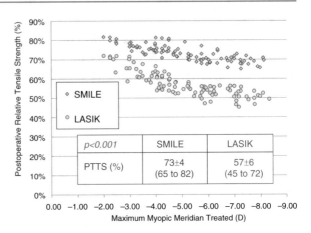

Fig. 13.8 Postoperative total tensile strength (as calculated by a previously published model [24]) plotted against maximum myopic meridian treated for a routine clinical population of SMILE cases and a population of LASIK cases matched for sphere, cylinder, and pachymetry. Despite a larger optical zone used in the SMILE group, the postoperative total tensile strength was still 16 % greater on average than in the LASIK group

p<0.001	SMILE	LASIK
PTTS (%)	73±4 (65 to 82)	57±6 (45 to 72)

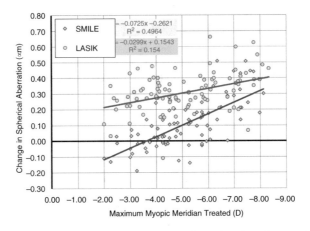

Fig. 13.9 Change in spherical aberration (OSA notation) plotted against maximum myopic meridian treated for a routine clinical population of SMILE cases and a population of LASIK cases matched for sphere, cylinder, and pachymetry. The greater postoperative total tensile strength after SMILE enabled the use of a larger optical zone in the SMILE group and consequently a lower induction of spherical aberration and therefore better optical quality than in the LASIK group

Figure 13.8 shows the postoperative total tensile strength calculated for all eyes using our model. Mean postoperative total tensile strength was 73 % (range 65–82 %) for the SMILE group and 57 % (range 45–72 %) for the LASIK group. Figure 13.9 shows the corneal spherical aberration induction (Atlas) for a 6 mm analysis zone for both groups. Mean change in spherical aberration (OSA notation) was 0.11 ± 0.16 μm (range −0.19 to 0.51 μm) for the SMILE group and 0.31 ± 0.12 μm (range −0.11 to 0.66 μm) for the LASIK group.

Measuring the biomechanical differences between SMILE and LASIK in vivo is a difficult challenge as currently there are very few instruments designed for this purpose. There are five studies where the Ocular Response Analyzer (Reichert Inc, Depew, NY) has been used to generate corneal hysteresis (CH) and corneal resistance factor (CRF), and all showed that CH and CRF were reduced after SMILE [34–38]. In two contralateral eye studies, CH and CRF were slightly greater after SMILE than LASIK [37, 38], while three other studies reported no difference in either CH or CRF between the SMILE and LASIK groups [34–36]. These results do not agree with the expected increased biomechanical strength after SMILE as described above. However, it is likely that CH and CRF are not ideal parameters for measuring corneal biomechanics [39] given that many studies show no change in CH and CRF after cross-linking [40]. It is also well known that CH and CRF are correlated with corneal pachymetry [41], so it would be expected for CH and CRF to be reduced after SMILE due to tissue removal.

Finally, there are two studies reporting the changes after SMILE and LASIK as measured using a Scheimpflug noncontact dynamic tonometer (Corvis ST) [28, 65]. Both studies found that the Corvis parameters were reduced after both procedures, but with no statistically significant difference between procedures. However, one study also found no difference between SMILE and LASEK [28].

13.3 Evidence for Other Biomechanical Changes After SMILE

Using the Artemis® very high-frequency digital ultrasound scanner (ArcScan Inc, Morrison, Colorado), we have also measured the accuracy of cap thickness and lenticule thickness achieved in SMILE. In a study including 70 eyes of 37 patients [42], the mean central cap thickness accuracy was found to be −0.7 µm (range −11 to +14 µm) for intended cap thicknesses over the range of 80–140 µm (i.e., the cap was on average 0.7 µm thinner than the intended cap thickness). The reproducibility of central cap thickness was found to be 4.4 µm [42]. In a second study in the same population [43], the readout central lenticule depth was 8.2 µm thicker on average than the Artemis measured stromal thickness change.

The systematic difference of 8 µm could be due to one of three reasons (or a combination of these): (1) an error in the VisuMax® cutting accuracy for one of the two layers, (2) error with the stromal change measurement by Artemis® VHF digital ultrasound, or (3) evidence for a biomechanical change in the stroma.

For there to be an error in the lenticule thickness due to VisuMax® cutting accuracy, there would have to be an error only in one of the interfaces. However, as described earlier, the cap thickness was accurate with a central accuracy of −0.7 µm [42]. Therefore, if the lenticule thickness difference was due to the VisuMax® cutting accuracy, the error must have been in the lower interface of the lenticule. However, the accuracy in our previous study was found to be similar for cap thicknesses between 80 and 140 µm [42], which provides evidence that the accuracy of the VisuMax® does not vary with depth (although this needs to be confirmed for depths at which the lower interface of the lenticule is created).

As with any measurement, there are always associated measurement errors. In this study, Artemis VHF digital ultrasound measurements of stromal thickness were made before and at least 3 months after surgery. This method eliminates the error induced by epithelial thickness changes that would be included with any full corneal thickness change method [42, 44]. The Artemis also has a very high repeatability for corneal (1.68 μm) and stromal (1.78 μm) thickness measurements, so this source of error was minimized [45]. In any event, errors such as these would be randomly distributed and would be likely to average out rather than result in a systematic error. Another source of error is the alignment between the two scans. In contrast to the other sources of measurement error, alignment error could be expected to be more likely to occur in one direction. As the corneal pachymetry is thinnest centrally and thicker radially toward the periphery, the lenticule is centered close to the thinnest point on the cornea in most cases unless the pachymetry is significantly decentered from the corneal vertex. Therefore, any misalignment in the postoperative scan will mean that the thinnest point of the postoperative scan will not be aligned with the thinnest point of the preoperative scan. This means that in the majority of cases, an alignment error will tend to underestimate the change in stromal thickness, as was observed in this population.

However, it is unlikely that these alignment errors could explain a systematic difference of 8 μm because the pachymetric progression of the central stroma is relatively gradual [46]. Therefore, the present study seems to provide evidence for some central stromal expansion caused by biomechanical changes occurring after SMILE. One possible mechanism could be that the lamellae severed by the lenticule *in between* the residual bed and the cap might be recoiling and causing expansion of the stroma as they are no longer under tension, similar to the known peripheral stromal expansion after LASIK [1, 4]. This expansion might be keeping the bottom lamellae of the cap slightly apart from the top lamellae of the residual bed. It seems unlikely that there would be any reason for the stroma in the residual bed or the cap to be expanding as they are still under tension. For example, the high accuracy of cap thickness that we have previously reported [42] provides evidence for biomechanical stability within the cap.

It is almost inevitable that there will be biomechanical changes after any corneal surgical procedure, so it is not surprising that there was a difference between the theoretical and achieved lenticule thickness. The fact that the difference was only 8 μm, of which a proportion can be explained by measurement error, implies that there is actually very little biomechanical change after SMILE, as might be expected given that only the stroma required is removed and that the strongest anterior stroma [7] and Bowman's layer [26] remain intact. This was also borne out in the results of the study as there was a lower degree of scatter in the SMILE lenticule thickness data compared with a similar result for excimer laser ablation depth in a LASIK population [44] indicating that there may have been a less variable biomechanical response after SMILE.

13.4 Ocular Surface and Corneal Sensitivity

The cornea is one of the most densely innervated peripheral tissues in humans. Nerve bundles within the anterior stroma grow radially inward from the periphery toward the central cornea [47, 48]. The nerves then penetrate Bowman's layer and create a dense network of nerve fibers, known as the subbasal nerve plexus, by branching both vertically and horizontally between Bowman's layer and basal epithelial cells. In LASIK, subbasal nerve bundles and superficial stromal nerve bundles in the flap interface are cut by the microkeratome or femtosecond laser, with only nerves entering the flap through the hinge region being spared. Subsequent excimer laser ablation severs further stromal nerve fiber bundles. Therefore, corneal sensitivity is decreased while the nerves regenerate. The lower corneal sensitivity can lead to a reduction in the blink rate, resulting in epitheliopathy (known as LASIK-induced neurotrophic epitheliopathy) due to the increased ocular surface exposure and patients feel "dry eye" [49, 50]. While there are also other contributing factors, it is generally accepted that corneal denervation is the largest factor [51–53].

Therefore, following the introduction of SMILE, there was an expectation that SMILE may demonstrate an improvement in postoperative dry eye compared to LASIK given that the anterior cornea is left untouched other than the small incision and the diameter of the cap is smaller than the diameter of a LASIK flap. While the trunk nerves that ascend into the epithelial layer within the diameter of the cap will still be severed in SMILE, those that ascend outside the cap diameter or that are anterior to the cap interface will be spared. A number of studies have investigated this by measuring corneal sensitivity [54–62] using esthesiometry and corneal innervation using confocal microscopy [57, 61, 63].

In our study including 156 eyes, corneal sensitivity was reduced in the early postoperative period after SMILE, but recovered to within 5 mm of baseline in 76 % of eyes by 3 months and in 89 % of eyes by 6 months [54]. In this study, we also performed a literature review of studies reporting the corneal sensitivity after LASIK and plotted our results against the average of the 21 LASIK studies. Our SMILE results compared favorably to LASIK with less reduction in central corneal sensitivity at all time points, particularly in the first 3 months.

Similar results have been reported in other SMILE studies. Wei et al. [55] found significantly higher central corneal sensitivity in the SMILE group ($n=61$) compared with the LASIK group ($n=54$) at 1 week, 1 month, and 3 months. Central corneal sensitivity decreased only slightly at 1 week and recovered to baseline 3 months after SMILE, whereas it had not reached baseline in the LASIK group. Similar results were found in a larger study by the same group [56].

Vestergaard et al. [57] performed a contralateral eye study comparing central corneal sensitivity after FLEx and SMILE in 35 myopic patients. At the 6-month time point, mean central corneal sensitivity was found to have returned to the baseline level in the SMILE group (1.0 mm less than baseline, $p>0.05$). In contrast, mean central corneal sensitivity was 3.8 mm less than baseline in the FLEx group ($p<0.05$) and was statistically significantly lower than the SMILE group.

Demirok et al. [58] performed a contralateral eye study comparing central corneal sensitivity after LASIK and SMILE in 28 myopic patients over a 6-month follow-up period. Mean central corneal sensitivity was reduced after both SMILE and LASIK at 1 week, 1 month, and 3 months; however, it was statistically significantly higher in the SMILE group at each of these time points. Central corneal sensitivity had returned to baseline levels at the 6-month time point in both groups.

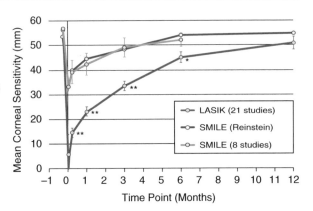

Fig. 13.10 Line graph showing the mean central corneal sensitivity over the 12-month follow-up period averaged across 8 SMILE studies and 21 LASIK studies following a review of the peer-reviewed literature

Although there was a difference in corneal sensitivity, other dry eye parameters were not affected including tear breakup time, Schirmer test, and tear film osmolarity.

Li et al. [59, 60] compared the change in central corneal sensitivity between SMILE ($n=38$) and LASIK ($n=31$) over a 6-month follow-up period. Mean central corneal sensitivity was reduced after both SMILE and LASIK at 1 week, 1 month, 3 months, and 6 months; however, it was statistically significantly higher in the SMILE group at each of these time points. As with the previous study, although there was a difference in corneal sensitivity, there were no real differences between groups for other dry eye parameters, such as tear breakup time, Schirmer test, and the Ocular Surface Disease Index (OSDI) questionnaire. Similar results were found by the same group in a second study [61].

Gao et al. [62] compared the change in central corneal sensitivity between SMILE ($n=30$) and LASIK ($n=64$) over a 3-month follow-up period. Mean central corneal sensitivity was reduced after SMILE at 1 week and 1 month, but had recovered to baseline by 3 months. The reduction in central corneal sensitivity after LASIK was significantly greater than after SMILE at all time points and was still 39 % lower than baseline at 3 months. This study also showed that SMILE resulted in milder ocular surface changes than LASIK in terms of fluorescein staining, tear breakup time, OSDI scores, IL-6 and NGF levels, and TNF-α and ICAM-1 concentrations.

Figure 13.10 shows the average corneal sensitivity (across all eight studies after SMILE) plotted over time [54–62]. For comparison, the graph also shows the average corneal sensitivity (across 21 studies [54] after LASIK where the Cochet-Bonnet esthesiometer had been used) plotted over time.

A few studies have also investigated the change in corneal innervation using confocal microscopy. Vestergaard et al. [57] demonstrated that the decrease in corneal nerves was greater after LASIK compared with SMILE at 6 months. Li et al. [61] found that the decrease in subbasal nerve fiber density was less severe in the first 3 months after SMILE than after LASIK. Similarly, Mohamed-Noriega et al.

found less nerve damage and faster nerve recovery in rabbit eyes 4 weeks after SMILE compared to LASIK [63]. A detailed review on this topic has been presented in Chap. 3 of this book.

Finally, a recent study by Xu et al. [64] compared dry eye parameters between SMILE and LASIK. They found that all parameters became worse in the early postoperative period in both groups; however, Schirmer test, tear breakup time, and the McMonnies score were all better in the SMILE group.

13.5 Summary

The evolution of SMILE, a flapless intrastromal keyhole keratomileusis procedure, has introduced a new method for corneal refractive surgery that minimizes the change in corneal biomechanics compared to PRK and LASIK by leaving the stronger anterior stroma intact. Despite SMILE lenticule profiles being essentially spherical, induction of spherical aberration in SMILE was lower than aspheric LASIK for equivalent or greater tissue removal. In preserving stronger anterior stromal lamellae, SMILE optical zones can be safely increased to improve spherical aberration control while still leaving postoperative relative corneal tensile strength higher than for an equivalent modern aspheric LASIK procedure. The other advantage of the flapless mechanism of SMILE is that there is greater preservation of the anterior corneal nerve plexus resulting in faster recovery of corneal innervation and corneal sensitivity.

References

1. Reinstein DZ, Silverman RH, Raevsky T, Simoni GJ, Lloyd HO, Najafi DJ, Rondeau MJ, Coleman DJ (2000) Arc-scanning very high-frequency digital ultrasound for 3D pachymetric mapping of the corneal epithelium and stroma in laser in situ keratomileusis. J Refract Surg 16(4):414–430
2. Dupps WJ Jr, Roberts C (2001) Effect of acute biomechanical changes on corneal curvature after photokeratectomy. J Refract Surg 17(6):658–669
3. Dupps WJ, Roberts C, Schoessler JP (1995) Peripheral lamellar relaxation. Paper presented at the ARVO 1995, Fort Lauderdale
4. Roberts C (2000) The cornea is not a piece of plastic. J Refract Surg 16(4):407–413
5. Knox Cartwright NE, Tyrer JR, Jaycock PD, Marshall J (2012) Effects of variation in depth and side cut angulations in LASIK and thin-flap LASIK using a femtosecond laser: a biomechanical study. J Refract Surg 28(6):419–425. doi:10.3928/1081597x-20120518-07
6. Medeiros FW, Sinha-Roy A, Alves MR, Dupps WJ Jr (2011) Biomechanical corneal changes induced by different flap thickness created by femtosecond laser. Clinics (Sao Paulo) 66(6): 1067–1071
7. Randleman JB, Dawson DG, Grossniklaus HE, McCarey BE, Edelhauser HF (2008) Depth-dependent cohesive tensile strength in human donor corneas: implications for refractive surgery. J Refract Surg 24(1):S85–S89
8. MacRae S, Rich L, Phillips D, Bedrossian R (1989) Diurnal variation in vision after radial keratotomy. Am J Ophthalmol 107(3):262–267

9. Maloney RK (1990) Effect of corneal hydration and intraocular pressure on keratometric power after experimental radial keratotomy. Ophthalmology 97(7):927–933

10. Muller LJ, Pels E, Vrensen GF (2001) The specific architecture of the anterior stroma accounts for maintenance of corneal curvature. Br J Ophthalmol 85(4):437–443

11. Ousley PJ, Terry MA (1996) Hydration effects on corneal topography. Arch Ophthalmol 114(2):181–185

12. Simon G, Ren Q (1994) Biomechanical behavior of the cornea and its response to radial keratotomy. J Refract Corneal Surg 10(3):343–351; discussion 351–346

13. Simon G, Small RH, Ren Q, Parel JM (1993) Effect of corneal hydration on Goldmann applanation tonometry and corneal topography. Refract Corneal Surg 9(2):110–117

14. Kohlhaas M, Spoerl E, Schilde T, Unger G, Wittig C, Pillunat LE (2006) Biomechanical evidence of the distribution of cross-links in corneas treated with riboflavin and ultraviolet A light. J Cataract Refract Surg 32(2):279–283. doi:10.1016/j.jcrs.2005.12.092

15. Scarcelli G, Pineda R, Yun SH (2012) Brillouin optical microscopy for corneal biomechanics. Invest Ophthalmol Vis Sci 53(1):185–190. doi:10.1167/iovs.11-8281

16. Petsche SJ, Chernyak D, Martiz J, Levenston ME, Pinsky PM (2012) Depth-dependent transverse shear properties of the human corneal stroma. Invest Ophthalmol Vis Sci 53(2):873–880. doi:10.1167/iovs.11-8611

17. Winkler M, Shoa G, Xie Y, Petsche SJ, Pinsky PM, Juhasz T, Brown DJ, Jester JV (2013) Three-dimensional distribution of transverse collagen fibers in the anterior human corneal stroma. Invest Ophthalmol Vis Sci 54(12):7293–7301. doi:10.1167/iovs.13-13150

18. Dawson DG, Grossniklaus HE, McCarey BE, Edelhauser HF (2008) Biomechanical and wound healing characteristics of corneas after excimer laser keratorefractive surgery: is there a difference between advanced surface ablation and sub-Bowman's keratomileusis? J Refract Surg 24(1):S90–S96

19. Roy AS, Dupps WJ Jr (2011) Patient-specific computational modeling of keratoconus progression and differential responses to collagen cross-linking. Invest Ophthalmol Vis Sci 52(12): 9174–9187. doi:10.1167/iovs.11-7395

20. Patel S (1987) Refractive index of the mammalian cornea and its influence during pachometry. Ophthalmic Physiol Opt 7(4):503–506

21. Kolozsvari L, Nogradi A, Hopp B, Bor Z (2002) UV absorbance of the human cornea in the 240- to 400-nm range. Invest Ophthalmol Vis Sci 43(7):2165–2168

22. Seiler T, Kriegerowski M, Schnoy N, Bende T (1990) Ablation rate of human corneal epithelium and Bowman's layer with the excimer laser (193 nm). Refract Corneal Surg 6(2):99–102

23. Huebscher HJ, Genth U, Seiler T (1996) Determination of excimer laser ablation rate of the human cornea using in vivo Scheimpflug videography. Invest Ophthalmol Vis Sci 37(1):42–46

24. Reinstein DZ, Archer TJ, Randleman JB (2013) Mathematical model to compare the relative tensile strength of the cornea after PRK, LASIK, and small incision lenticule extraction. J Refract Surg 29(7):454–460. doi:10.3928/1081597x-20130617-03

25. Schmack I, Dawson DG, McCarey BE, Waring GO 3rd, Grossniklaus HE, Edelhauser HF (2005) Cohesive tensile strength of human LASIK wounds with histologic, ultrastructural, and clinical correlations. J Refract Surg 21(5):433–445

26. Seiler T, Matallana M, Sendler S, Bende T (1992) Does Bowman's layer determine the biomechanical properties of the cornea? Refract Corneal Surg 8(2):139–142

27. Sinha Roy A, Dupps WJ, Jr., Roberts CJ (2014) Comparison of biomechanical effects of small-incision lenticule extraction and laser in situ keratomileusis: finite-element analysis. J Cataract Refract Surg. 40:971–980

28. Shen Y, Chen Z, Knorz MC, Li M, Zhao J, Zhou X (2014) Comparison of corneal deformation parameters after SMILE, LASEK, and femtosecond laser-assisted LASIK. J Refract Surg. 30(5):310–318

29. Reinstein DZ, Archer TJ, Gobbe M (2011) LASIK for myopic astigmatism and presbyopia using non-linear aspheric micro-monovision with the carl zeiss meditec MEL 80 platform. J Refract Surg 27(1):23–37

30. Ganesh S, Gupta R (2014) Comparison of visual and refractive outcomes following femtosecond laser- assisted lasik with smile in patients with myopia or myopic astigmatism. J Refract Surg 30(9):590–596

31. Lin F, Xu Y, Yang Y (2014) Comparison of the visual results after SMILE and femtosecond laser-assisted LASIK for myopia. J Refract Surg 30(4):248–254. doi:10.3928/1081597x-20140320-03

32. Agca A, Demirok A, Cankaya KI, Yasa D, Demircan A, Yildirim Y, Ozkaya A, Yilmaz OF (2014) Comparison of visual acuity and higher-order aberrations after femtosecond lenticule extraction and small-incision lenticule extraction. Cont Lens Anterior Eye. doi:10.1016/j.clae.2014.03.001

33. Reinstein DZ, Archer TJ, Gobbe M (2014) ReLEx SMILE induces significantly less spherical aberration than wavefront optimised sub-Bowman's LASIK for any given residual postoperative relative tensile strength. Paper presented at the ARVO 2014, Orlando

34. Vestergaard AH, Grauslund J, Ivarsen AR, Hjortdal JO (2014) Central corneal sublayer pachymetry and biomechanical properties after refractive femtosecond lenticule extraction. J Refract Surg 30(2):102–108. doi:10.3928/1081597-20140120-05

35. Agca A, Ozgurhan EB, Demirok A, Bozkurt E, Celik U, Ozkaya A, Cankaya I, Yilmaz OF (2014) Comparison of corneal hysteresis and corneal resistance factor after small incision lenticule extraction and femtosecond laser-assisted LASIK: a prospective fellow eye study. Cont Lens Anterior Eye 37(2):77–80. doi:10.1016/j.clae.2013.05.003

36. Kamiya K, Shimizu K, Igarashi A, Kobashi H, Sato N, Ishii R (2014) Intraindividual comparison of changes in corneal biomechanical parameters after femtosecond lenticule extraction and small-incision lenticule extraction. J Cataract Refract Surg 40(6):963–970. doi:10.1016/j.jcrs.2013.12.013

37. Wu D, Wang Y, Zhang L, Wei S, Tang X (2014) Corneal biomechanical effects: Small-incision lenticule extraction versus femtosecond laser-assisted laser in situ keratomileusis. J Cataract Refract Surg 40(6):954–962. doi:10.1016/j.jcrs.2013.07.056

38. Wang D, Liu M, Chen Y, Zhang X, Xu Y, Wang J, To CH, Liu Q (2014) Differences in the corneal biomechanical changes after SMILE and LASIK. J Refract Surg 30(10):702–707. doi:10.3928/1081597x-20140903-09

39. Reinstein DZ, Gobbe M, Archer TJ (2011) Ocular biomechanics: measurement parameters and terminology. J Refract Surg 27(6):396–397

40. Goldich Y, Barkana Y, Morad Y, Hartstein M, Avni I, Zadok D (2009) Can we measure corneal biomechanical changes after collagen cross-linking in eyes with keratoconus?–a pilot study. Cornea 28(5):498–502

41. Touboul D, Roberts C, Kerautret J, Garra C, Maurice-Tison S, Saubusse E, Colin J (2008) Correlations between corneal hysteresis, intraocular pressure, and corneal central pachymetry. J Cataract Refract Surg 34(4):616–622

42. Reinstein DZ, Archer TJ, Gobbe M (2013) Accuracy and reproducibility of cap thickness in small incision lenticule extraction. J Refract Surg 29(12):810–815. doi:10.3928/1081597x-20131023-02

43. Reinstein DZ, Archer TJ, Gobbe M (2014) Lenticule thickness readout for small incision lenticule extraction compared to artemis three-dimensional very high-frequency digital ultrasound stromal measurements. J Refract Surg 30(5):304–309

44. Reinstein DZ, Archer TJ, Gobbe M (2010) Corneal ablation depth readout of the MEL80 excimer laser compared to artemis three-dimensional very high-frequency digital ultrasound stromal measurements. J Refract Surg 26(12):949–959

45. Reinstein DZ, Archer TJ, Gobbe M, Silverman RH, Coleman DJ (2010) Repeatability of layered corneal pachymetry with the artemis very high-frequency digital ultrasound arc-scanner. J Refract Surg 26(9):646–659

46. Reinstein DZ, Archer TJ, Gobbe M, Silverman R, Coleman DJ (2009) Stromal thickness in the normal cornea: three-dimensional display with artemis very high-frequency digital ultrasound. J Refract Surg 25(9):776–786

47. He J, Bazan NG, Bazan HE (2010) Mapping the entire human corneal nerve architecture. Exp Eye Res 91(4):513–523. doi:10.1016/j.exer.2010.07.007

48. Tuisku IS, Lindbohm N, Wilson SE, Tervo TM (2007) Dry eye and corneal sensitivity after high myopic LASIK. J Refract Surg 23(4):338–342
49. Wilson SE (2001) Laser in situ keratomileusis-induced (presumed) neurotrophic epitheliopathy. Ophthalmology 108(6):1082–1087
50. Savini G, Barboni P, Zanini M, Tseng SC (2004) Ocular surface changes in laser in situ keratomileusis-induced neurotrophic epitheliopathy. J Refract Surg 20(6):803–809
51. Solomon R, Donnenfeld ED, Perry HD (2004) The effects of LASIK on the ocular surface. Ocul Surf 2(1):34–44
52. Shtein RM (2011) Post-LASIK dry eye. Expert Rev Ophthalmol 6(5):575–582. doi:10.1586/eop.11.56
53. Chao C, Golebiowski B, Stapleton F (2014) The role of corneal innervation in LASIK-induced neuropathic dry eye. Ocul Surf 12(1):32–45. doi:10.1016/j.jtos.2013.09.001
54. Reinstein DZ, Archer TJ, Gobbe M, Bartoli E (2014) Corneal sensitivity after small incision lenticule extraction (SMILE). J Cataract Refract Surg (in press)
55. Wei S, Wang Y (2013) Comparison of corneal sensitivity between FS-LASIK and femtosecond lenticule extraction (ReLEx flex) or small-incision lenticule extraction (ReLEx smile) for myopic eyes. Graefes Arch Clin Exp Ophthalmol 251(6):1645–1654. doi:10.1007/s00417-013-2272-0
56. Wei SS, Wang Y, Geng WL, Jin Y, Zuo T, Wang L, Wu D (2013) Early outcomes of corneal sensitivity changes after small incision lenticule extraction and femtosecond lenticule extraction. Zhonghua Yan Ke Za Zhi 49(4):299–304
57. Vestergaard AH, Gronbech KT, Grauslund J, Ivarsen AR, Hjortdal JO (2013) Subbasal nerve morphology, corneal sensation, and tear film evaluation after refractive femtosecond laser lenticule extraction. Graefes Arch Clin Exp Ophthalmol 251(11):2591–2600. doi:10.1007/s00417-013-2400-x
58. Demirok A, Ozgurhan EB, Agca A, Kara N, Bozkurt E, Cankaya KI, Yilmaz OF (2013) Corneal sensation after corneal refractive surgery with small incision lenticule extraction. Optom Vis Sci 90(10):1040–1047. doi:10.1097/OPX.0b013e31829d9926
59. Li M, Zhao J, Shen Y, Li T, He L, Xu H, Yu Y, Zhou X (2013) Comparison of dry eye and corneal sensitivity between small incision lenticule extraction and femtosecond LASIK for myopia. PLoS One 8(10):e77797. doi:10.1371/journal.pone.0077797
60. Li M, Zhou Z, Shen Y, Knorz MC, Gong L, Zhou X (2014) Comparison of corneal sensation between small incision lenticule extraction (SMILE) and femtosecond laser-assisted LASIK for myopia. J Refract Surg 30(2):94–100. doi:10.3928/1081597x-20140120-04
61. Li M, Niu L, Qin B, Zhou Z, Ni K, Le Q, Xiang J, Wei A, Ma W, Zhou X (2013) Confocal comparison of corneal reinnervation after small incision lenticule extraction (SMILE) and femtosecond laser in situ keratomileusis (FS-LASIK). PLoS One 8(12), e81435. doi:10.1371/journal.pone.0081435
62. Gao S, Li S, Liu L, Wang Y, Ding H, Li L, Zhong X (2014) Early changes in ocular surface and tear inflammatory mediators after small-incision lenticule extraction and femtosecond laser-assisted laser in situ keratomileusis. PLoS One 9(9), e107370. doi:10.1371/journal.pone.0107370
63. Mohamed-Noriega K, Riau AK, Lwin NC, Chaurasia SS, Tan DT, Mehta JS (2014) Early corneal nerve damage and recovery following small incision lenticule extraction (SMILE) and laser in situ keratomileusis (LASIK). Invest Ophthalmol Vis Sci 55(3):1823–1834. doi:10.1167/iovs.13-13324
64. Xu Y, Yang Y (2014) Dry eye after small incision lenticule extraction and LASIK for myopia. J Refract Surg 30(3):186–190. doi:10.3928/1081597x-20140219-02
65. Pedersen IB, Bak-Nielsen S, Vestergaard AH, Ivarsen A, Hjortdal J (2014) Corneal biomechanical properties after LASIK, ReLEx flex, and ReLEx smile by Scheimpflug-based dynamic tonometry. Graefes Arch Clin Exp Ophthalmol 252(8):1329–1335

Centration in SMILE for Myopia

14

Apostolos Lazaridis and Walter Sekundo

Contents

The centration of the treatment zone during corneal refractive procedures remains a topic of great dispute among refractive surgeons. Despite the benefits of a pupillary centration [1, 2], it is widely accepted that a centration in regard to the visual axis [3, 4] is the key to optimized visual outcomes while maintaining the functional corneal morphology after the treatment. The advent of eye trackers led to a significant reduction of extended decentrations and therefore to fewer functional deficits, such as reduced corrected distance visual acuity, irregular astigmatism, halos, glare [5], reduced contrast sensitivity [6], and monocular diplopia [7]. However, despite the efficacy of laser treatments based on eye-tracking systems, the problem of subclinical decentrations (<1.0 mm) and the induction of higher-order aberrations (HOAs) still remain [8].

Financial Disclosure The authors have no financial interest in any topics related to this study. Prof. Dr. med. Walter Sekundo is a member of the scientific board of Carl Zeiss Meditec AG

A. Lazaridis (✉)
Department of Ophthalmology, Philipps University of Marburg, Marburg, Germany
e-mail: aposlaz_bsn@hotmail.com

W. Sekundo
Department of Ophthalmology, Philipps University of Marburg and Universitätsklinikum Giessen & Marburg GmbH, Marburg, Germany

© Springer International Publishing Switzerland 2015
W. Sekundo (ed.), *Small Incision Lenticule Extraction (SMILE): Principles, Techniques, Complication Management, and Future Concepts*, DOI 10.1007/978-3-319-18530-9_14

14.1   Intraoperative Alignment in SMILE

Unlike excimer laser procedures, where the alignment of the photoablation can be adjusted by the surgeon (objective alignment) and is controlled by eye trackers, in all-in-one femtosecond procedures like femtosecond lenticule extraction (FLEx) and small incision lenticule extraction (SMILE) [9–11], the alignment of the photo-disruption is subjective and relies entirely on the patient, who must fixate on a blinking light during the suction process and during the initial stage of the laser scan (after the laser cut of the lenticule's posterior plane, the blinking target is obscured by intracorneal gas bubbles). The surgeon controls and encourages the patient to maintain fixation in particular, when the patient's view is obscured by intrastromal gas bubbles during the second half of the laser procedure in order to avoid suction loss. In SMILE for myopia correction, the centration is targeted at the corneal vertex (CV), which is identified by the coaxially sighted corneal light reflex (CSCLR) or the first image of Purkinje.

The issue of centration in SMILE and other corneal refractive procedures for myopia correction is considered to be less critical compared to hyperopic treatments. Due to the small or moderate degree of angle kappa in myopic eyes and the larger optical zone of the treated areas, centering the procedure on the CSCLR results on similar refractive and visual outcomes as targeting at the entrance pupil center (EPC). However, determining the patterns of the achieved centration on such cases would help us coordinate the centration on hyperopic or high myopic eyes with larger angle K. This chapter presents a centration analysis of the treatment zone on myopic eyes with small or moderate angle K treated with SMILE and evaluates the predictability of the intraoperative alignment and its pattern in regard to the visual axis.

14.2   Targeting at the Coaxially Sighted Corneal Light Reflex

Refractive lenticule extractions and standard ablation profiles can effectively correct myopia and myopic astigmatism. However, the quality of vision in many cases could decrease substantially, especially under mesopic and low-contrast conditions [12, 13], due to induction of HOAs, even by subclinical decentrations as small as 0.2 mm [8]. Several researchers including Uozato and Guyton [1] back in 1987 supported the opinion that corneal refractive procedures should be centered at the EPC rather than the CSCLR. Indeed, a centration targeted at the EPC allows the whole aperture of the eye's optical system to be covered with the ablation profile [1, 2] and minimizes the required optical zone. In addition, the EPC can be easily located and tracked by eye-tracking systems. This could potentially eliminate the risk of extended decentrations or nonhomogenous ablation patterns. However, the pupil center is an unstable point which shifts with changes in pupil diameter [14], and the entrance pupil, used as reference point, is a virtual image of the real pupil as seen through the cornea. Moreover, the efficacy of pupil tracking might be limited due to parallax error because the eye tracker locates corneal positions by tracking the subjacent EPC [15, 16].

In contrast, the CSCLR provides stable morphologic reference, which in cases of small or moderate angle K is considered a good approximation of the point where the visual axis intersects the cornea, offering the opportunity of maintaining the functional corneal morphology after surgery. Many studies have reported outcomes in favor of the centration at the CSCLR. Pande and Hillman [3] proposed the CSCLR as the reference point for an ideal centration closest to the CV. Arbelaez et al. [12] showed no significant differences regarding the visual and refractive outcomes between CV and pupil centration. Nevertheless, fewer HOAs were induced after centering the refractive procedure on the CV. Kermani et al. [17] reported a greater risk of decentered ablations and inducted HOAs by hyperopic treatments centered on the line of sight. CSCLR is increasingly regarded as the preferable reference point of centration regardless of the degree of angle K. Reinstein et al. [4] presented in 2013 a major study comparing refractive outcomes, visual quality, and subjective night vision between two groups of eyes with small and large angle kappa after moderate to high hyperopic LASIK where the ablation was centered on the CSCLR. The results showed similar outcomes in both groups for all tested parameters, providing evidence that refractive corneal ablation should not be systematically aligned with the EPC. A problem, however, that could arise by the centration on the CSCLR is that determining its exact location depends on the surgeon's eye dominance, the surgeon's eye balance, or the stereopsis angle of the microscope [12, 18].

In order to evaluate the predictability of the subjective intraoperative alignment in SMILE and assess the pattern of the achieved centration in regard to the visual axis, we conducted a centration study on myopic eyes with small or moderate angle K, with the centration being targeted at the CSCLR. All procedures were performed by a single surgeon using the VisuMax® platform (Carl Zeiss Meditec AG/Germany). The measurements were performed on the pachymetry maps of Pentacam™ (Oculus, Germany). Patient and surgical data are presented in Tables 14.1 and 14.2. The findings are presented in the following subsections.

Table 14.1 Patient data

Groups	Patients	Gender (M/F)	Total eyes OD/OS	Age	SEQ (Dpt)	Cylinder (Dpt)
SMILE	36	16/20	34/35	38±10 (22–55)	−5.96±1.9 (−1.25 to −10)	−0.95±1.0 (0 to −4.0)

[a]*SEQ* spherical equivalent, *Dpt* diopter
[b]Descriptive statistics (i.e., average, standard deviation, minimum, maximum, and range) were performed using Microsoft Excel 2010 (Microsoft Corporation, Redmond, WA)

Table 14.2 Surgical data

Groups	SEQ of the correction (Dpt)	Cylinder of the correction (Dpt)	Flap/cap thickness (μm)	Flap/cap diameter (mm)	Lenticule thickness/ ablation depth (μm)	Lenticule/ ablation diameter (mm)
SMILE	−5.70±1.95 (−1.25 to −10)	−0.79±1.04 (0 to −4.0)	118±3.8 (100–120)	7.8±0.1 (7.5–8.0)	120±27 (48–164)	6.7±0.2 (6.2–7.0)

[a]*SEQ* spherical equivalent, *Dpt* diopter
[b]Descriptive statistics (i.e., average, standard deviation, minimum, maximum, and range) were performed using Microsoft Excel 2010 (Microsoft Corporation, Redmond, WA)

14.3   Angle K and the Pattern of the Achieved Centration

A very important issue regarding the achieved centration is its pattern in regard to the visual axis. The visual axis is the line which connects the fovea with the fixation point via the nodal point of the eye. The line of sight is defined as the line connecting the fixation point with the center of the entrance pupil. The pupillary axis is the line passing through the EPC perpendicular to the cornea. The definition of angle kappa (angle K) is the angular distance between visual and pupillary axis [19–21], which is in myopic eyes approximately 2.0° and is mostly positive [19, 22]. As a result of positive angle K the first image of Purkinje is located nasal to the pupillary center or temporal in cases of a negative angle K. Studies conducted in order to assess the distribution of angle K in myopic eyes showed a prevalence of positive angle K in the majority of the tested subjects, while a negative angle K or no angle K was identified in substantially less cases [19, 23].

For our study purposes the degree of angle K was estimated indirectly by the coordinates of the CV on the preoperative pachymetry maps of Pentacam. When the patient fixates on the red spot, in the middle of the monochromatic slit light source (blue LED at 475 nm), then the reference axis of the instrument (measurement axis) and the patient's visual axis would be coaxial. In this case the intercept of the instrument's reference axis and the cornea would be the CV [19, 24]. This point is called corneal apex (CA) in the Pentacam software, which is a misnomer for vertex [19, 25], as the CA should academically refer to the point of greatest corneal curvature or shortest radius [24] (Fig. 14.1). Knowing the location of the CV, we can estimate the location of the preoperative CSCLR and also evaluate the angle K, because the CSCLR is a good approximation of the point where the visual axis intersects the cornea.

In order to assess the angle K of the examined eyes, the points corresponding to the preoperative CSCLR were depicted on a Cartesian system in relation to the EPC

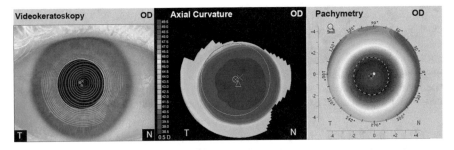

Fig. 14.1 Corneal landmarks as being identified by Altas (Carl Zeiss Meditec AG, Germany) and Pentacam™ (Oculus, Germany) for the same patient. The first two images (videokeratoskopy and axial curvature) were created by Atlas. The corneal vertex (CV) is depicted with an X, the entrance pupil center (EPC) with ⊗ and the corneal apex (CA) with △. The last image represents a postoperative pachymetry map of Pentacam. The EPC is depicted with a cross, the pupil edge with a white dotted circle and the CA with a white dot. Note that the point identified as CA by Pentacam has the same displacement in relation to the EPC as the CV on Atlas images. This example further supports the observation that the CA in Pentacam software is actually the CV

(Fig. 14.2). Regarding the angle K of the right eyes (blue dots), the points with positive x-coordinates correspond to positive angle K, while the points having negative x-coordinates correspond to negative angle K. Regarding the angle K of the left eyes (red dots), the points with negative x-coordinates correspond to positive angle K, while the points with positive x-coordinates correspond to negative angle K. When the points were located on the y-axis (0, y), the angle K was 0°. The preoperative CSCLR demonstrated a nasalization pattern, since in most eyes angle K was positive. The mean distance of the preoperative CSCLR from the EPC was 0.227±0.121, ranging from 0.014 to 0.602.

In order to evaluate the pattern of the achieved centration in regard to the visual axis, we located on each eye the coordinates of the point of maximum pachymetrical difference (PMPD) on the differential pachymetry maps and depicted it on a Cartesian system in relation to the EPC (Fig. 14.3). The PMPD corresponds to the maximum refractive power and the center of mass of the lenticule and therefore represents the achieved centration. The results were compared to the preoperative pattern of the CSCLR in relation to the EPC (Fig. 14.2). We examined for each eye the displacement of the PMPD on the x-axis in relation to the preoperative CSCLR. The achieved centration would follow the pattern of angle K if the x-coordinate of the PMPD maintained the same sign (+ or −) as the x-coordinate of the preoperative CSCLR. We concluded that 26 out of 34 right eyes (76.47 %) and

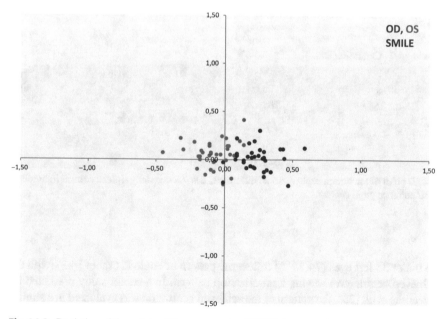

Fig. 14.2 Depiction of the points of the preoperative CSCLR (attempted centration) in relation to the EPC (0,0) in SMILE group. The degree of angle K could be evaluated by the location of the preoperative CSCLR, because the CSCLR is a good approximation of the point where the visual axis intersects the cornea

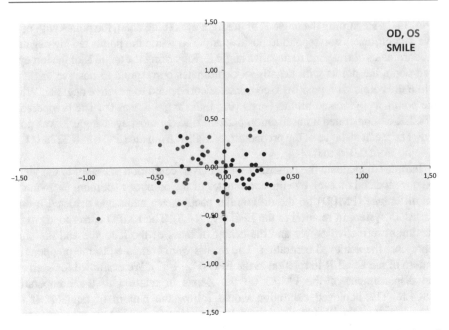

Fig. 14.3   Achieved Centration after SMILE in relation to EPC (0,0). Note that the distribution of the points, which represent the achieved centration, follows the preoperative pattern of angle K (Fig. 14.2)

Table 14.3   Centration data

Group	Mean distance between PMPD and preoperative CSCLR (mm)	Preoperative pattern of angle K (no. of eyes)			Achieved centration following the preoperative pattern of angle K
		Pos	Neg	None	
SMILE	0.315±0.211	OD	32	2	0	26/34 (76.47 %)
	(0.0 to −1.131)	OS	24	11	0	26/35 (74.28 %)
		Total	56	13	0	52/69 (75.36 %)

PMPD point of maximum pachymetrical difference, *CSCLR* coaxially sighted corneal light reflex, *EPC* entrance pupil center

26 out of 35 left eyes (74.28 %) follow the pattern of angle K (Table 14.3), with the achieved centration showing a nasalization pattern. In a recent study presented by Lazaridis et al. [26], the pattern of the achieved centration was evaluated in a similar group of patients treated with femtosecond laser assisted-LASIK (FS-LASIK). In that case the reference point of centration was the EPC. The results showed a random distribution pattern of the achieved centration in regard to the visual axis (Figs. 14.4 and 14.5).

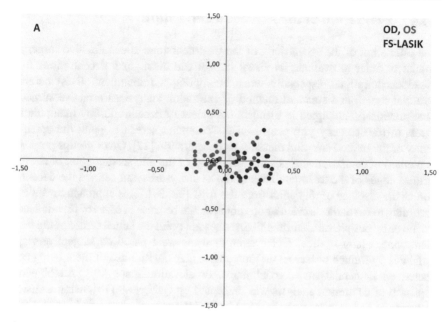

Fig. 14.4 Depiction of the points of the preoperative CSCLR in relation to the EPC (0,0) in FS-LASIK group (Data from publication of Lazaridis et al. [26])

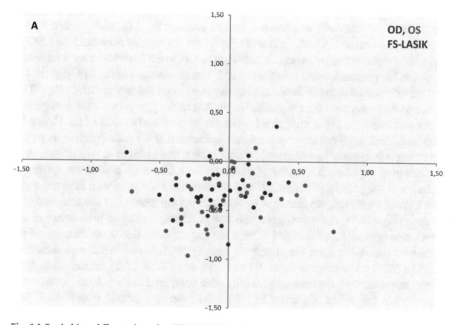

Fig. 14.5 Achieved Centration after FS-LASIK in relation to EPC (0,0). A centration analysis was performed on a group FS-LASIK treated eyes, similar to the group of SMILE treated eyes presented in this chapter. The alignment was targeted at the EPC. Note the random distribution of the centers of the treatment zones in regard to the preoperative pattern of angle K (Fig. 14.4) (Data from publication of Lazaridis et al. [26])

14.4   Evaluation of the Achieved Centration

The estimation of the eccentricity of the treatment zone after refractive surgery is crucial in order to evaluate its visual impact and distinguish decentrations from pseudodecentrations, especially when attempting a retreatment. It is therefore essential to define a standard method of centration analysis. Refractive surgeons have previously attempted to estimate the extent of decentration by manipulating sheets of transparency film placed on the computer screen to point the apparent center of the treated area and measure its decentration [27]. Other groups proposed as method of centration analysis the estimation of the intersecting point of the four farthest edges of the treatment zone in the x- and y-axes and defined the decentration as the distance of this point from the EPC [28, 29]. This approach however is according to the author's calculations not accurate because in cases of pseudodecentration or by peripheral abnormalities, it does not point the actual center of the treatment zone. Many studies of centration analysis were based on subjective visual estimates by trained observers on topography maps, with most of them being conducted on tangential maps, axial maps, or elevation maps [30]. An objective approach of centration analysis was presented by Qazi et al. [15], using a custom software on Orbscan topography in order to determine the topographic functional optical zone and the centroid of this zone on refractive maps.

The centration analysis described in this chapter was performed on the differential pachymetry maps of Pentacam. The point of maximum pachymetrical difference (PMPD), which corresponds to the maximum refractive power and the center of mass of the lenticule, was located, and its distance from the topographical pupil center and from the CA was measured (Fig. 14.6). As already explained the CSCLR would be represented by the coordinates of the CA when the instrument's reference axis and the patient's visual axis are coaxial. The coordinates of the EPC and the CA on the differential maps of Pentacam are the same as on the preoperative maps. That allowed us to evaluate the centration in relation to the preoperative corneal parameters and therefore avoid misguided measurements related to shift of the CA or the topographical pupil center, which might be observed at the postoperative maps due to changes in corneal morphology, corneal optics, and changes in pupil diameter.

Bringing together the PMPD of each eye on a Cartesian coordinate system in relation to the preoperative CSCLR and marking the right eyes with blue color and the left eyes with red, we managed to visualize the attempted and the achieved centration (Fig. 14.7). As we observe, the points corresponding to the centers of the lenticules are quite accumulated around the target point. The mean distance of the achieved centration from the attempted target (CSCLR) in SMILE was measured 0.315 ± 0.211 mm, ranging from 0.0 to 1.131 mm (Table 14.3). In the study from Lazaridis et al. [26], the centration results were compared to FS-LASIK. Despite the eye-tracker controlled alignment in FS-LASIK, the eyes treated with SMILE presented better centration results, with the decentration in FS-LASIK being measured 0.452 ± 0.224 mm, ranging from 0.02 to 1.040 mm. The incidence of small

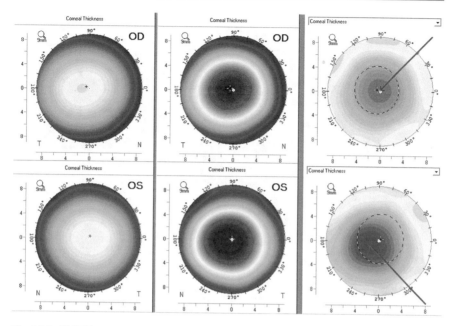

Fig. 14.6 SMILE case - Pachymetry maps of the same patient preoperative, 3 months postoperative and differential pachymetry maps. The EPC is depicted with a cross, the pupil edge with a *white dotted circle* and the CA with a white dot. The *red arrow* shows the point of the maximum pachymetrical difference. Right eye (OD): well centered lenticule zone (distance of the thickest point from CA: 0.103 mm, distance of the thickest point from EPC: 0.243 mm). Left eye (OS): decentered lenticule zone (distance of the thickest point from CA: 0.863 mm, distance of the thickest point from EPC: 1.062 mm)

(0–0.2 mm), moderate (0.2–0.5 mm), and high (0.5–1 mm or >1 mm) decentrations was also estimated. As presented in Table 14.4, there were 24 eyes with small, subclinical decentrations up to 0.2 mm, 32 eyes with moderate decentrations up to 0.5 mm, and only 13 cases with higher decentrations (0.5–1 mm or >1 mm). Compared to FS-LASIK, Lazaridis et al. [26] reported significantly more FS-LASIK eyes with highly decentered ablation profiles (histogram Fig. 14.8). Another centration analysis in SMILE was presented by Li et al. [31], with the eccentricity of the treatment zone being measured by a Scheimpflug-based system. The author of this study reported a mean decentered displacement of 0.17 ± 0.09 mm. The decentered displacement of all treated eyes (100) was within 0.50 mm, while 70 eyes were within 0.20 mm and 90 eyes were within 0.30 mm.

The differential pachymetry maps used for the centration analysis provided a very good depiction of the treatment zone, and moreover, the centroid of this zone corresponded to the point of the maximum pachymetrical difference and therefore the center of mass of the lenticule, regardless of the extent of decentration [26]. On the differential tangential maps however, in cases of extended decentrations or

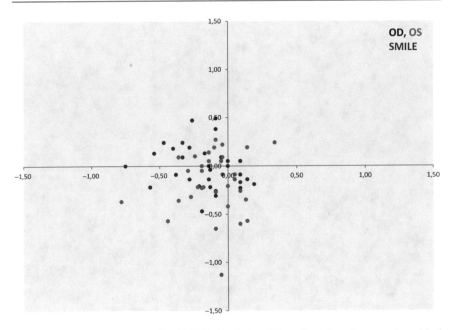

Fig. 14.7 Achieved Centration after SMILE - Depiction of the points of maximum pachymetrical difference in relation to the preoperative CSCLR (0,0). Note that points representing the achieved centration are more accumulated around the target point (CSCLR) compared to the achieved centration after FS-LASIK (Fig. 14.5)

Table 14.4 Extend of decentration in SMILE

Decentration	0–0.2 mm	0.2–0.5 mm	0.5–1 mm	>1 mm
No. of SMILE eyes	24/69 (34.78 %)	32/69 (46.38 %)	12/69 (17.39 %)	1/69 (1.45 %)

peripheral abnormalities, the center of the treatment zone was not that well depicted. Moreover, in these cases the point of the maximum diopter difference did not correspond to the center of the treatment zone. According to the literature, the center of the treatment zone on tangential differential maps is defined as the centroid of the area with a refractive power of 1.0 diopter more than the zero refractive power obtained from the differential map [8]. In the SMILE case demonstrated in Fig. 14.9, that would be the area inside the yellow-orange ring. The tangential maps would be the most appropriate maps to use in order to evaluate the refractive effect of

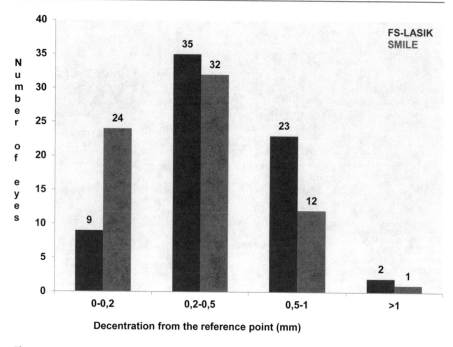

Fig. 14.8 Histogram of the distance of the points of maximum pachymetrical difference from the reference point of its technique (mm). SMILE eyes are presented with red columns and FS-LASIK eyes with blue (Data from publication of Lazaridis et al. [26])

decentration, estimate the degree of peripheral abnormalities, or determine the edge of the treatment zone [30]. The same problem is observed on the differential axial maps. In this case the visual assessment of the centroid of the treatment zone is even more challenging due to the tendency of the axial algorithm to ignore minor variations in curvature [30]. Visual estimations of the center of the treatment zone on the differential elevation maps are also difficult because of the poor resolution setting. Tangential, axial, and elevation maps could be used in cases of a well-centered treatment zone with well-defined edges in order to visually identify its centroid. However, in cases of sizable decentrations, it was difficult to visually estimate the center of the treatment zone on other maps rather than the differential pachymetry maps (Fig. 14.9). Furthermore, they provide three-dimensional data (pachymetry data correspond to z-axis) despite the two-dimensional display, which is crucial in order to fully assess the centration of three-dimensional objects such as lenticules.

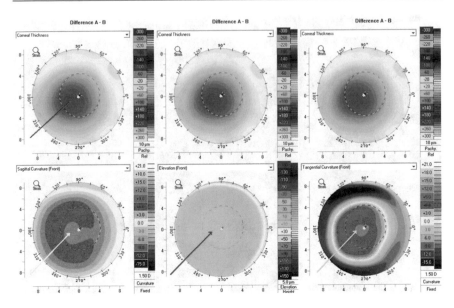

Fig. 14.9 SMILE case of extended decentration - Distance of the thickest point from CA: 0.863 mm. Distance of the thickest point from EPC: 1.062 mm. With the Pentacam software when we place the cursor at one point on the pachymetry maps we get same point depicted on all other maps. Note that a visual estimation of the center of the treatment zone is easier on the differential pachymetry maps. The corneal thickness, as measured by Pentacam, is the distance between the anterior and posterior corneal surface, measured normal to the anterior surface tangent. This approach is commonly used for assessing the volume of the lenticule or the ablation and their spatial distribution in the corneal stroma. Moreover, the pachymetry maps despite being projected on a two-dimensional display, they provide sufficient three-dimentional data (pachymetry corresponds to z-axis) and they generate reliable subtraction maps, provided that both pre- and postoperative measurements are well aligned. On the subtraction maps, the pachymetry progression from the periphery to the thickest point demonstrates the actual volume of the extracted lenticule or the photoablated tissue as well as its center

14.5 Summary

The subjective alignment in SMILE has raised the argument that a good centration could not be guaranteed due to the absence of eye trackers. According to published data, in SMILE we do achieve a good centration [26, 31] which in most cases follows the preoperative pattern of angle K [26]. Furthermore, since the photodisruption is performed under suction, once we obtain a good centration, we can maintain it throughout the whole laser procedure. Finally, the intraoperative alignment targeted at the CSCLR results to a more natural centration, closer to the visual axis as compared to the alignment at the EPC [26].

References

1. Uozato H, Guyton DL (1987) Centering corneal surgical procedures. Am J Ophthalmol 103:264–275
2. Soler V, Benito A, Soler P et al (2011) A randomized comparison of pupil-centered versus vertex-centered ablation in LASIK correction of hyperopia. Am J Ophthalmol 152:591–599
3. Pande M, Hillman JS (1993) Optical zone centration in keratorefractive surgery: entrance pupil center, visual axis, coaxially sighted corneal reflex, or geometric corneal center? Ophthalmology 100:1230–1237
4. Reinstein DZ, Gobbe M, Archer TJ (2013) Coaxially sighted corneal light reflex versus entrance pupil center centration of moderate to high hyperopic corneal ablations in eyes with small and large angle kappa. J Refract Surg 29(8):518–525
5. Fay AM, Trokel SL, Myers JA (1992) Pupil diameter and the principal ray. J Cataract Refract Surg 18(4):348–351
6. Terrell J, Bechara SJ, Nesburn A, Waring GO, Macy J, Maloney RK (1995) The effect of globe fixation on ablation zone centration in photorefractive keratectomy. Am J Ophthalmol 119(5):612–619
7. Mulhern MG, Foley-Nolan A, O'Keefe M, Condon PI (1997) Topographical analysis of ablation centration after excimer laser photorefractive keratectomy and laser in situ keratomileusis for high myopia. J Cataract Refract Surg 23(4):488–494
8. Mrochen M, Kaemmerer M, Mierdel P, Seiler T (2001) Increased higher-order optical aberrations after laser refractive surgery: a problem of subclinical decentration. J Cataract Refract Surg 27(3):362–369
9. Sekundo W, Kunert K, Russmann C, Gille A, Bissmann W, Stobrawa G, Sticker M, Bischoff M, Blum M (2008) First efficacy and safety study of femtosecond lenticule extraction for the correction of myopia: six-month results. J Cataract Refract Surg 34(9):1513–1520
10. Blum M, Kunert K, Schröder M, Sekundo W (2010) Femtosecond lenticule extraction for the correction of myopia: preliminary 6-month results. Graefes Arch Clin Exp Ophthalmol 248(7):1019–1027
11. Sekundo W, Kunert KS, Blum M (2011) Small incision corneal refractive surgery using the small incision lenticule extraction (SMILE) procedure for the correction of myopia and myopic astigmatism: results of a 6 month prospective study. Br J Ophthalmol 95(3):335–339
12. Arbelaez MC, Vidal C, Arba-Mosquera S (2008) Clinical outcomes of corneal vertex versus central pupil references with aberration-free ablation strategies and LASIK. Invest Ophthalmol Vis Sci 49(12):5287–5294
13. Mastropasqua L, Toto L, Zuppardi E, Nubile M, Carpineto P, Di Nicola M, Ballone E (2006) Photorefractive keratectomy with aspheric profile of ablation versus conventional photorefractive keratectomy for myopia correction: six-month controlled clinical trial. J Cataract Refract Surg 32(1):109–116
14. Yang Y, Thompson K, Burns S (2002) Pupil location under mesopic, photopic and pharmacologically dilated conditions. Invest Ophthalmol Vis Sci 43(7):2508–2512
15. Qazi MA, Pepose JS, Sanderson JP, Mahmoud AM, Roberts CJ (2009) Novel objective method for comparing ablation centration with and without pupil tracking following myopic laser in situ keratomileusis using the bausch & lomb technolas 217A. Cornea 28(6):616–625
16. Bueeler M, Mrochen M (2004) Limitations of pupil tracking in refractive surgery: systematic error in determination of corneal locations. J Refract Surg 20(4):371–378
17. Kermani O, Oberheide U, Schmiedt K, Gerten G, Bains HS (2009) Outcomes of hyperopic LASIK with the NIDEK NAVEX platform centered on the visual axis or line of sight. J Refract Surg 25:98–103

18. de Ortueta D, ArbaMosquera S (2007) Centration during hyperopic LASIK using the coaxial light reflex. J Refract Surg 23(1):11
19. Park CY, Oh SY, Chuck RS (2012) Measurement of angle kappa and centration in refractive surgery. Curr Opin Ophthalmol 23(4):269–275
20. Tabernero J, Benito A, Alcon E, Artal P (2007) Mechanism of compensation of aberrations in the human eye. J Opt Soc Am A Opt Image Sci Vis 24(10):3274–3283
21. Basmak H, Sahin A, Yildirim N, Papakostas TD, Kanellopoulos AJ (2007) Measurement of angle kappa with synoptophore and Orbscan II in normal population. J Refract Surg 23(5): 456–460
22. Von Noorden G, Campos E (2002) Examination of the patient II. In: Binocular vision and ocular motility-theory and management of strabismus, 6th edn. Mosby, St. Louis, pp 168–173
23. Scott WE, Mash AJ (1973) Kappa angle measures of strabismic and nonstrabismic individuals. Arch Ophthalmol 89(1):18–20
24. Mandell RB, Chiang CS, Klein SA (1995) Location of the major corneal reference points. Optom Vis Sci 72(11):776–784
25. Xu J, Bao J, Lu F, He JC (2012) An indirect method to compare the reference centres for corneal measurements. Ophthalmic Physiol Opt 32(2):125–132
26. Lazaridis A, Droutsas K, Sekundo W (2014) Topographic analysis of the centration of the treatment zone after SMILE for myopia and comparison to FS-LASIK: subjective versus objective alignment. J Refract Surg 30(10):680–686
27. Deitz MR, Piebenga LW, Matta CS, Tauber J, Anello RD, DeLuca M (1996) Ablation zone centration after photorefractive keratectomy and its effect on visual outcome. J Cataract Refract Surg 22(6):696–701
28. Azar DT, Yeh PC (1997) Corneal topographic evaluation of decentration in photorefractive keratectomy: treatment displacement vs. intraoperative drift. Am J Ophthalmol 124(3): 312–320
29. Lin DT, Sutton HF, Berman M (1993) Corneal topography following excimer photorefractive keratectomy for myopia. J Cataract Refract Surg 19(Suppl):149–154
30. Vinciguerra P, Randazzo A, Albè E, Epstein D (2007) Tangential topography corneal map to diagnose laser treatment decentration. J Refract Surg 23(9 Suppl):S1057–S1064
31. Li M, Zhao J, Miao H, Shen Y, Sun L, Tian M, Wadium E, Zhou X (2014) Mild decentration measured by a Scheimpflug camera and its impact on visual quality following SMILE in the early learning curve. Invest Ophthalmol Vis Sci 55(6):3886–3892

How to Improve the Refractive Predictability of SMILE

15

Jesper Hjortdal, Anders Vestergaard, and Anders Ivarsen

Contents

15.1   Introduction

Small-incision lenticule extraction (ReLEx® SMILE) has been developed as a corneal refractive flap-free procedure in which an intrastromal lenticule is cut by a femtosecond laser and manually extracted through a peripheral corneal tunnel incision [9]. It is anticipated that the procedure will reduce some of the potential side effects of LASIK, such as eye dryness, epithelial ingrowth at the flap edge, a long-term risk for traumatic flap dislocation [11] and corneal ectasia which may develop during the years after surgery (Toda 2008). In the published studies so far, the refractive predictability, safety and patient satisfaction of ReLEx smile are high and comparable to Fs-LASIK [1, 4].

J. Hjortdal, MD, PhD, DMSc (✉) • A. Vestergaard, MD, PhD • A. Ivarsen, MD, PhD
Department of Ophthalmology, Aarhus University Hospital, Aarhus, Denmark
e-mail: jesper.hjortdal@dadlnet.dk

© Springer International Publishing Switzerland 2015
W. Sekundo (ed.), *Small Incision Lenticule Extraction (SMILE)*:
Principles, Techniques, Complication Management, and Future Concepts,
DOI 10.1007/978-3-319-18530-9_15

This chapter will present and discuss theoretical and empirical considerations on how to further optimise the refractive predictability of the SMILE procedure. The theoretical limits for subjective refractive predictability will be addressed, aspects of actual lenticule cutting and dissection will be discussed, the importance of biological variations in corneal wound healing will be considered, and finally, possible individual factors affecting refractive predictability will be evaluated empirically using a cohort of 1,800 eyes treated by SMILE for moderate and high myopia.

15.2 Theoretical Limits for Spherical Equivalent Refractive Predictability

The spherical equivalent (SE) refractive predictability is usually evaluated by calculating the difference between the attempted change in refraction and the achieved change in subjective refraction. The attempted change is the difference between the preoperative subjective SE refraction and the SE target refraction, and these values are entered in the femtosecond laser. The achieved change in refraction is calculated as the postoperative subjective SE refraction subtracted by the preoperative subjective refraction. Thus, the refractive predictability, or the error in the surgical correction, is identical to the difference between the SE target refraction and the postoperative SE subjective refraction. Overcorrections will be positive in value, and undercorrections will be negative. The average error for a group of eyes is the accuracy, while the standard deviation on this error for a group of eyes describes the precision of the procedure. Repeatability conditions are when replicate measurements are made in one setting, by a single observer, using the same equipment over a short time period. A common definition of reproducibility conditions is when different observers, working in different clinics, make the replicate measurements using different equipment over an extended time period.

15.3 Variations in Subjective Refraction

It is well known that clinical subjective refraction has a certain variation. If the same patient is refracted twice, the difference between these repeated refractions would have some scatter although no intervention has taken place. The actual variation in repeated clinical refraction in eyes with no surgical intervention has been studied in detail [7, 10]. The standard deviation on the SE difference between two clinical refractions has been found to be between 0.22 and 0.40 dioptres. Lower values are typically found when the same optometrist or surgeon undertakes measurements twice in the same clinic using the same equipment and following the same protocol (intraobserver repeatability), while higher values are observed if different and unrelated observers are performing the measurements in the same clinic using the same equipment (interobserver repeatability), and even higher if measurements are performed in different clinics using different equipment (interobserver reproducibility).

Most surgeons will agree that clinical refraction tends to be slightly less precise in eyes that have been treated with corneal refractive surgery, possibly due to an increase in optical higher-order aberrations. It has, however, not been possible to identify repeatability studies on clinical subjective refraction in eyes that have undergone corneal refractive laser procedures.

Thus, taking into account that the predictability of a procedure is based on two clinical refractions, the theoretical lowest precision of, for example, a SMILE procedure will be between 0.22 and 0.40 dioptres but possibly slightly higher due to a "softer" subjective refraction in postoperative laser-treated eyes.

The actual prediction error in femtosecond laser refractive surgery can be decomposed into errors caused by variations in clinical refraction (0.22–0.40 diopters), errors caused by variation in actual laser cutting of the lenticule and errors caused by a variation in the biomechanical response or wound healing response between eyes and individual patients.

15.4 Variations in Lenticule Cutting

In SMILE surgery, the cap thickness is theoretically constant across the anterior lenticule cut, while the attempted refractive correction is achieved by varying the posterior lenticule cut. Studies have shown that the cap thickness can be created accurately and with a precision (SD) of between 5 and 11 μm [6, 12, 14] and an average within eye cap thickness of around 4.3 μm. Variations in cap thickness can influence the refractive reproducibility if there is a systematic change from centre to periphery. If the cap thickness is higher than intended in the periphery, a larger refractive effect will be achieved, and vice versa, while scattered variations will have no systematic effect.

A single published study has addressed and compared the actual attempted central lenticule thickness with measurements of changes in stromal thickness measured by very high-frequency ultrasound (Artemis, more on this issue see Chap. 13) [8]. On average, the VisuMax® read-out lenticule depth was 8.2 ± 8.0 μm thicker (range: −8 to +29 μm) than the Artemis measured stromal change. A proportion of this difference may be real but can also be caused by alignment errors or changes in ultrasound velocity in the cornea caused by the procedure.

We have analysed original data from our prospective, randomised study of ReLEx® FLEX and SMILE in a contralateral eye study [12, 13]. Thirty-five patients were treated for moderate to high myopia with FLEX in one eye and SMILE in the other. Optical low-coherence reflectometry (Haag Streit, Switzerland) was used to measure central corneal thickness (CCT) before and 6 months after surgery. From the measurements, the net reduction in CCT could be calculated and compared with the VisuMax® read-out of central lenticule thickness.

The analyses showed that the net reduction in CCT was 22.9 ± 6.6 μm less than expected in the FLEX operated eyes and 21.5 ± 6.4 μm less than expected in SMILE-operated eyes. This apparent error in net corneal thickness reduction was compared with the individual spherical equivalent prediction error by correlation analysis.

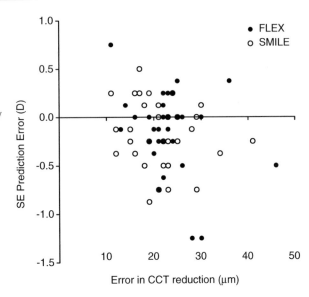

Fig. 15.1 Plot of the spherical equivalent prediction error (D) by the difference in central corneal thickness between the expected (VisuMax read-out lenticule thickness) and the observed change measured by optical low-coherence tomography

There was, however, no significant correlation between these parameters (Fig. 15.1). This finding suggests that errors in lenticule cutting resulting in less decrease in CCT do not influence the refractive predictability of a ReLEx procedure. Thus, only systematic gradual errors from centre to periphery will affect the ultimate change in SE refractive power.

The mechanism of femtosecond laser cutting may affect the refractive precision of the SMILE procedure [2]. At the laser focus point, the laser energy increases above a critical level, and plasma formation and cavitation take place. The actual point of focus is associated with some degree of imprecision that is determined by lateral and axial beam scanning imprecision. However, the axial point of interaction between laser pulse and corneal tissue may fluctuate due to non-linear effects within a certain range that is approximately given by the Rayleigh length (z_R) (Fig. 15.2).

The VisuMax® femtosecond laser operates with a wavelength of 1,043 nm (λ) and a beam waist (w_0) of 1 µm. The beam waist is dependent on a number of optical factors related to the femtosecond laser system. From the known parameters, the Rayleigh length can be calculated to be about 3 µm. This shows that the axial position of individual points of interaction is stable within a range of about 3 µm. The VisuMax technology fulfils the applicative requirements if it is taken into account that the cut surface is defined by millions of adjacent points of interactions, and the cap will function as a sort of low-pass filter to level out variations in the cut surfaces.

Sometimes the Rayleigh length is discussed in relation to the central profile thickness for a 1-diopter correction that is approximately 13 µm for a 6-mm diameter optical zone. However, from the previous considerations, this is misleading, because the relevant parameter to observe is the overall change in corneal curvature and not the central profile thickness. Further optimisation of the femtosecond laser

Fig. 15.2 The actual point of focus of the femtosecond laser is associated with some degree of imprecision and is characterised by the Rayleigh length (z_R). The Rayleigh length is dependent on the wavelength (λ) and the beam waist (w_0). (Courtesy: Dirk Mühlhoff, Carl Zeiss Meditec AG, Jena, Germany)

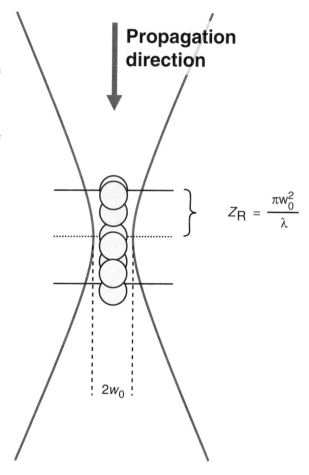

$$z_R = \frac{\pi w_0^2}{\lambda}$$

with respect to wavelength and beam waist is discussed today. If the wavelength could be reduced to one-third and/or the beam waist could be lowered further, the Rayleigh length would be reduced. However, it is questionable whether such technological modifications would actually be useful and are at all possible.

15.5   Biological Variations

15.5.1 Epithelium

From basic studies of excimer laser refractive procedures, it is known that compensatory wound healing takes place after surgery. In photorefractive surgery, stromal remodelling and new synthesis of collagen, which is laid down on the bared stroma, can affect the refractive reproducibility. After PRK and LASIK for myopia, considerable thickening of the central epithelium takes place, and this will also reduce the net refractive effect of the procedures. Up to a 10 µm increase in central epithelium has been documented by confocal microscopy over time after correction for approximately 7 diopters of myopia [3]. This is acknowledged as a result of the normal beneficial smoothing effect of the epithelium to reduce abrupt changes in the stromal surface shape. After SMILE, central epithelial thickening have also been documented by optical coherence tomography, but the thickening amounted to only 6 µm on average with considerable variation between eyes (range −2 to 13 µm) [12]. Using very high-frequency ultrasound, epithelial thickening of 15 µm has, however, been observed after SMILE [8]. A 6-µm increase in epithelial thickness corresponds to a regression of approximately 0.4 dioptres. Some of the variation in epithelial thickness changes is caused by measurement inaccuracy. However, individual differences between patients and eyes concerning epithelial hyperplasia undoubtedly are a major contributor to variations in refractive predictability after SMILE. Compared with LASIK, the effective optical zone is larger after SMILE, and this possibly explains that compensatory epithelial thickening is less after SMILE.

15.5.2 Biomechanics

In SMILE, the majority of the anterior lamellae are preserved compared to the anatomical situations after LASIK, and as such, the SMILE-operated cornea is more biomechanically intact compared with the post-LASIK cornea. Mathematical simulations have confirmed this ([5], Chap. 13). The effect of individual variations in corneal biomechanics and susceptibility to development of corneal ectasia, in theory, should be less in SMILE compared with LASIK-treated eyes. Today, corneal ectasia development after SMILE has not been published although more than 100,000 procedures have been performed worldwide. Overall, it is fair to expect that individual variations in corneal biomechanical properties are less prone to affect refractive predictability after SMILE compared with LASIK.

15.5.3 Empirical Studies of Factors Affecting the Refractive Predictability of SMILE

In 2012, we published a paper on predictors for the outcome of SMILE [1]. Three hundred thirty-five patients with myopia up to 10 diopters (spherical equivalent refraction) and astigmatism up to 2 diopters were treated with small-incision lenticule extraction in both eyes (670 eyes) and followed for 3 months. The preoperative spherical equivalent averaged −7.19 D ± 1.30 D. In eyes with emmetropia as target refraction, 84.0 % obtained an uncorrected distance visual acuity ≤0.10 (logMAR) at 3 months. Mean corrected distance visual acuity improved from −0.03 to −0.05 (logMAR) ($p < 0.01$). 2.4 % (16 eyes) lost two or more lines of corrected distance visual acuity. The achieved refraction was 0.25 ± 0.44 D less than attempted after 3 months, and 80.1 % (537 eyes) and 94.2 % (631 eyes) were within ±0.5 and ±1.0

diopters of attempted, respectively. Multiple linear regression analyses revealed that spherical equivalent undercorrection was predicted by increasing patient age (0.1 D per decade; $p < 0.01$) and steeper corneal curvature (0.04 D per D; $p < 0.01$). The safety and efficacy of the procedure were minimally affected by age, gender, and simultaneous cylinder correction. In conclusion, the findings of an undercorrection of 0.25 diopters and small effects of patient age and corneal curvature suggest that the standard nomogram for SMILE needs only minor adjustments. However, this conclusion is related to a standard cup thickness (up to 130 μm) only. As stated in Chap. 12, thicker caps (or deeper lenticules) might need some adjustments in refractive data entered into the laser.

Here, we now extend the study to include more than 1,500 eyes treated for myopia with SMILE at Department of Ophthalmology, Aarhus University Hospital. The cohort of patients is the same as described by Ivarsen et al. [4]. After a thorough preoperative evaluation by trained optometrists, patients were thoroughly informed about keratorefractive surgery, including known side effects and complications.

From January 2011 to March 2013, 1,800 eyes of 922 consecutive patients were operated with SMILE at the Department of Ophthalmology, Aarhus University Hospital, Denmark. Patients were seen the day after surgery and again after 3 months; however, only 808 patients (1,574 eyes) attended the 3-month follow-up visit. The average preoperative patient characteristics are given in Table 15.1.

Patients underwent SMILE treatment by the VisuMax® femtosecond laser. At the 12-o'clock position, a 30–60° incision was created for lenticule extraction. Lenticule diameter ranged from 6.0 to 7.0 mm, and the lenticule side cut was 15 μm in all cases. Cap diameter varied from 7.3 to 7.7 mm, and the intended cap thickness was 110–130 μm. All cases were operated with one of two different laser energy settings. Setting 1 used a laser cut energy index of 25–27 (~130 nJ) and a spot spacing of 2.5–3.0 μm. In setting 2, a laser cut energy index of 34 (~170 nJ) and a spot spacing of 4.5 μm were used. Laser setting 1 was used for surgery in 656 eyes, and setting 2 was used in 1,144 procedures. After the laser treatment, a blunt spatula was used to break any remaining tissue bridges, allowing the lenticule to be removed with a pair of forceps. After removal of the lenticule, the stromal pocket was flushed

Table 15.1 Pre-operative demographics of 1,800 eyes treated with SMILE for myopia

	All eyes ($n = 1,800$)
Gender (male/female)	1,102/698
Age (yrs)	38 ± 8 (19–59)
Sphere (D)	−6.79 ± 1.99 (−14.25 to +1.75)
Cylinder (D)	−0.93 ± 0.90 (−5.75 to 0.00)
Spherical equivalent refraction (D)	−7.25 ± 1.84 (−14.50 to −0.25)
Keratometry (D)	43.27 ± 1.47 (38.93–48.35)
Central corneal thickness (μm)	535 ± 27.7 (473–634)
Intraocular pressure (mmHg)	15.2 ± 2.8 (7–24)

Values are given as mean ± standard deviation, with range in parentheses

with saline, and patients received 1 drop of chloramphenicol and 1 drop of diclofenac.

Postoperative treatment comprised fluorometholone and chloramphenicol eye drops four times daily for 1 week followed by two times per day the second week. The use of additional lubricating eye drops was encouraged. Three months after surgery, patients received a full clinical examination, including automated keratometry, Pentacam HR, manifest refraction, determination of uncorrected and corrected distance visual acuity.

Statistical analyses included unpaired t-tests (dichotomous variables), ANOVA (trichotomous variables), bivariate correlation analysis (continuous variables) and multiple linear regression analyses for evaluation of the effect of possible predictors for the outcome parameter predictability, which were assumed to follow a normal distribution. The effect of patient age and gender, eye (right/left), corneal curvature and central thickness, and attempted change in spherical equivalent refraction was analysed as independent variables. In addition, the two femtosecond laser settings were studied to determine whether they influenced the outcome parameters. Statistical analyses were performed in SPSS version 11 (SPSS Inc, Chicago, Illinois). Only variables with a significant ($P < 0.05$) bivariate correlation (continuous variables) or significant unpaired t-test or ANOVA test results (di- or trichotomous variables) were included in the multiple linear regression analysis (stepwise model with inclusion criteria: $P < 0.05$ and exclusion criteria: $P > 0.10$).

The achieved and attempted spherical equivalent corrections were highly correlated (R^2 . 0.94; $P < 0.01$) (Fig. 15.3a), with a mean postoperative refraction of -0.28 ± 0.52 D and a mean error in treatment of -0.15 ± -0.50 D (range, -2.00 to $+2.25$ D; Fig. 15.1). The dependency between the error in treatment and the attempted refractive change was significant ($R^2 = 0.044$, $P < 0.01$) (see Fig. 15.3b).

The results of the bivariate analyses on the effect of predictors for predictability, safety and efficacy are summarised in Table 15.2. The error in spherical equivalent refraction at 3 months after surgery was significantly influenced by patient age, gender, eye (right or left), corneal power, lenticule diameter, energy settings and experience (time).

The results of the multiple linear regression analysis are shown in Table 15.3. The model could only explain 5.0 % of the total variation in the error in spherical equivalent refraction at 3 months. Attempted refractive correction was the most important predictor amounting to a 6 % undercorrection. Patient age influenced the prediction error by undercorrection of 0.006 D per increasing year of age. Increasing preoperative corneal power influenced the refractive outcome by an undercorrection of 0.039 D per diopter of corneal steepening. Female gender was significantly predictive for an undercorrection of 0.085 D, and right eyes were undercorrected 0.09 dioptres compared with left eyes.

Fig. 15.3 (**a**) Achieved (3 months after surgery) versus attempted change in spherical equivalent refraction in +1,500 eyes treated with small-incision lenticule extraction (SMILE). Correlation coefficient and linear regression results are shown. Line of identity is also shown. (**b**) Error in spherical equivalent refraction (attempted subtracted by achieved change). Correlation coefficient and linear regression results are shown. Regression line is also shown

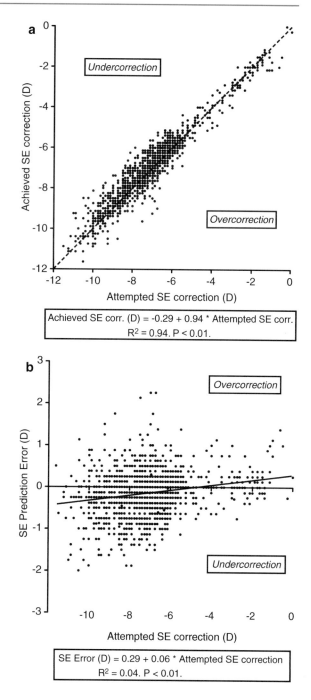

Achieved SE corr. (D) = -0.29 + 0.94 * Attempted SE corr.
$R^2 = 0.94$. $P < 0.01$.

SE Error (D) = 0.29 + 0.06 * Attempted SE correction
$R^2 = 0.04$. $P < 0.01$.

Table 15.2 Bivariate analysis of factors influencing the refractive outcome of SMILE for myopia

Bivariate analysis	Mean or R	SD	N	P
Gender (male/females)	−0.058/−0.196	0.458/0.512	575/978	<0.001
Eye (right/left)	−0.185/−0.105	0.477/0.512	777/776	0.002
Lenticule diameter (mm) (<6.00/6.00–6.50/>6.50)	−0.281/−0.130/−0.085	0.594/0.488/0.392	210/1,168/174	<0.001
Energy (1/2)	−0.109/−0.167	0.491/0.500	594/959	0.026
Time (Days)	−0.074		1,553	<0.01
Age (years)	−0.076		1,553	<0.01
Attempted correction (D)	0.212		1,553	<0.01
CCT (μm)	0.028		1,553	0.27
Keratometry (D)	−0.154		1,553	P<0.01

Means and standard deviations (SD) on prediction error for grouped variables (gender, eye, lenticule diameter, energy settings) and Pearson correlation coefficients (R) for time after SMILE surgery were initiated at Aarhus University Hospital, patient age, preoperative central corneal thickness (CCT) and keratometry. Statistical significance (P) for unpaired t-tests or ANOVA for di- or trichotomous variables or for significance of Pearson's correlation coefficient for continuous variables

Table 15.3 Multivariate analysis of factors influencing the refractive outcome of SMILE for myopia

Multivariate analysis	Coefficient	SEM	P
Gender (males)	0.085	0.0260	<0.001
Eye (right)	−0.087	0.0241	<0.001
Age (yrs)	−0.006	0.0015	<0.001
Attempted correction (D)	0.058	0.0081	<0.001
Keratometry (D)	−0.039	0.0086	<0.001

Results (coefficient and standard error (SEM)) from multiple linear regression analysis of possible predictors for the spherical equivalent prediction error after SMILE

15.6 Discussion

SMILE surgery for moderate and high myopia is, compared with our experience with microkeratome-based LASIK and femtosecond laser-based LASIK, more accurate and precise. In this chapter various sources of variation contributing to variation in the clinical refractive outcome have been presented. Novel results from the largest empirical study to date on predictors for the refractive outcome of SMILE documents that only 5 % of the variation in the refractive outcome after SMILE can be explained by demographic, biometric and identifiable surgical factors.

From the original analysis presented here, it appears that although the prediction error in SMILE appears fairly independent of the attempted correction, there seems to be a small, but significant increasing undercorrection with increasing refractive correction attempt. In the present study, all eyes operated at our department were included, while a previous study only included eyes treated for myopia up to −10 dioptres in SE refraction and only included eyes with low astigmatism (less than 2 dioptres) and uncomplicated surgery. The larger number of eyes included in the present study possibly adds to the finding of a significant effect of treatment attempt.

In the present study, the small but significant influence of increasing age, gender and corneal curvature corresponded to the previous study. A small, but significant effect of which eye was operated was, however, noted. Right eyes were 0.1 dioptres under-corrected compared with left eyes. The influence of the predictors was, however, very small, and with the exception of attempted correction, we do not suggest that these findings are used for nomogram adjustment. For attempted correction, it may be considered to decrease the attempted correction by 0.25 for low corrections (−1 to −2 dioptres) and to increase the attempted correction by 0.25 dioptres for high corrections (−8 and above).

Ninety-five percent of the variation in the SE prediction error could not be explained in the present study. The total standard deviation on the prediction error was 0.50 dioptres, corresponding to a variance of 0.25 dioptres^2. Considering that clinical refractions may be associated with a standard deviation of 0.4 dioptres, corresponding to a variance of 0.16 dioptres^2, and that empirical factors related to age, gender, eye, corneal power and treatment attempt explain 0.05 dioptres^2, only 0.04 dioptres^2 of the variance need to be explained. This amounts to a standard deviation of 0.2 dioptres on the prediction error. Further optimisation of the femto-second laser may be able to reduce the prediction error, but the majority of remaining errors possibly is related to individual differences in the compensatory epithelial hyperplasia.

It seems reasonable to believe that the most important factor to improve the refractive predictability of the SMILE procedure is very standardised protocols for the preoperative refractive evaluation of patients, preferably by repeated measurements of clinical refraction before surgery is planned.

References

1. Hjortdal J, Vestergaard A, Ivarsen A et al (2012) Predictors for the outcome of small-incision lenticule extraction for Myopia. J Refract Surg 28(12):865–871
2. Hjortdal J, Ivarsen A (2014) Corneal refractive surgery: is intracorneal the way to go and what are the needs for technology? Proc. SPIE 8930, Ophthalmic Technologies XXIV, 89300B (28 Feb 2014), doi:10.1117/12.2054449
3. Ivarsen A, Hjortdal J (2012) Seven-year changes in corneal power and aberrations after PRK or LASIK. Invest Ophthalmol Vis Sci 53(10):6011–6016
4. Ivarsen A, Asp S, Hjortdal J (2014) Safety and complications of more than 1500 small-incision lenticule extraction procedures. Ophthalmology 121(4):822–828
5. Reinstein D, Archer T, Randleman J (2013) Mathematical model to compare the relative tensile strength of the cornea after PRK, LASIK, and small incision lenticule extraction. J Refract Surg 29(7):454–460
6. Reinstein DZ, Archer TJ, Gobbe M (2013) Accuracy and reproducibility of cap thickness in small incision lenticule extraction. J Refract Surg 29(12):810–815
7. Reinstein DZ, Yap TE, Carp GI, Archer TJ, Gobbe M, London Vision Clinic optometric group (2014) Reproducibility of manifest refraction between surgeons and optometrists in a clinical refractive surgery practice. J Cataract Refract Surg 40(3):450–9
8. Reinstein DZ, Archer TJ, Gobbe M (2014) Lenticule thickness readout for small incision lenticule extraction compared to Artemis three-dimensional very high-frequency digital ultrasound stromal measurements. J Refract Surg 30(5):304–309

9. Sekundo W, Kunert K, Russmann C et al (2008) First efficacy and safety study of femtosecond lenticule extraction for the correction of myopia: six month results. J Cataract Refract Surg 34(9):1513–1520
10. Shah R, Edgar DF, Rabbetts R, Harle DE, Evans BJW (2009) Standardized patient methodology to assess refractive error reproducibility. Optom Vis Sci 86:517–528
11. Shah R, Shah S, Sengupta S (2011) Results of small incision lenticule extraction: all-in-one femtosecond laser refractive surgery. J Cataract Refract Surg 37(1):127–137
12. Vestergaard A, Grauslund J, Ivarsen A et al (2014) Central corneal sublayer pachymetry and biomechanical properties after refractive femtosecond lenticule extraction. J Refract Surg 30(2):102–108
13. Vestergaard A, Grauslund J, Ivarsen A et al (2014) Efficacy, safety, predictability, contrast sensitivity, and aberrations after femtosecond laser lenticule extraction. J Cataract Refract Surg 40(3):403–411
14. Zhao J, Yao P, Li M, Chen Z, Shen Y, Zhao Z, Zhou Z, Zhou X (2013) The morphology of corneal cap and its relation to refractive outcomes in femtosecond laser small incision lenticule extraction (SMILE) with anterior segment optical coherence tomography observation. PLoS One 8(8):e70208

Evaluating Corneal Cut Surface Quality in SMILE

16

Jon Dishler, Noël M. Ziebarth, Gregory J.R. Spooner, Jesper Hjortdal, and Sonia H. Yoo

Content

Creating high-quality corneal cuts in clinically acceptable treatment times has been a critical aspect of femtosecond laser corneal refractive surgery since its introduction in the late 1990s [1]. Considerable effort has gone into establishing laser-scanning designs, laser-scanning parameters, scanning patterns, and surgical techniques to produce the high-quality flaps, keratoplasties, and other femtosecond laser incisions that are in widespread use today. The surface quality of femtosecond laser cuts has

J. Dishler (✉)
Dishler Laser Institute, 8400 East Prentice Avenue, Suite 1200,
Greenwood Village, CO, USA
e-mail: jond@dishler.com

N.M. Ziebarth
Biomedical Atomic Force Microscopy Laboratory, Department of Biomedical Engineering,
University of Miami College of Engineering, 1251 Memorial Drive,
McArthur Annex Room 209, Coral Gables, FL, USA

G.J.R. Spooner
Gain Consulting Services, 129 Winfield Street, San Francisco, CA, USA

J. Hjortdal
Department of Clinical Medicine, Ophthalmology at Àarhus University Hospital, Ojenafd. J,
Norrebregade 44, bygn. 10.2., 8000 Àarhus C, Àarhus, Denmark
e-mail: jesper.hjortdal@dadlnet.dk

S.H. Yoo
Bascom Palmer Eye Institute, University of Miami Miller School of Medicine,
900 NW 17th Street, Miami, FL, USA

© Springer International Publishing Switzerland 2015   169
W. Sekundo (ed.), *Small Incision Lenticule Extraction (SMILE):*
Principles, Techniques, Complication Management, and Future Concepts,
DOI 10.1007/978-3-319-18530-9_16

steadily improved over the earliest instruments in which energies of several micro-joules and spot spacings on the order of 10 μm were used [1]. Faster and more accurate scanning systems, smaller laser focal spots, and lower energies have been the driving technological force enabling the trends of higher-quality cut surfaces and minimal opaque bubble layer (OBL) effects. As flap generation performed with the femtosecond laser keratome was perfected, lamellar resection quality approached [2] and then equaled the quality of resections produced by mechanical blades [3].

In the case of flaps and keratoplasties, the effort to improve femtosecond laser cutting and cut surface qualities was undertaken initially because the separation of cut tissue planes was required to be as good as those produced by mechanical blades. The effort to improve femtosecond laser cut quality continued as superior tissue dissection was believed to be associated with better corneal optical quality, a diminished inflammatory response, faster visual recovery, [2–7], and reduced TLSS [8].

A long-standing objective has been to produce direct refractive corrections to the cornea using ultrashort pulses lasers. Early attempts to develop intrastromal procedures included the use of picosecond lasers [9] and femtosecond lasers [1]. Today femtosecond lasers are used to produce direct refractive effects by changing the biomechanical strength of the cornea by relaxing incisions [10]. Until recently, the speed, quality, and control of scanned femtosecond lasers were insufficient to be used in a direct refractive procedure. There are three reasons for this limitation: (1) Cutting and removing a stromal tissue volume of the correct shape for a refractive correction must be made with precise and custom curvatures, as opposed to the disk-shaped cuts that were associated with earlier attempts to perform femtosecond keratomileusis [1]. (2) The lenticule to be removed must be freed from cut surfaces without direct access of the resected tissue under a lifted flap. (3) The block of tissue to be removed has a thin edge, typically between 10 and 30 μm, which is thinner than corneal flap or keratoplasty tissue margins. Corneal cut quality may therefore be more important in direct refractive procedures, such as SMILE and FLEX, or refractive implants that depend on femtosecond cut features, such as the KAMRA inlay, than it is for more established femtosecond procedures [11].

Femtosecond laser cut quality has generally followed a path towards smaller laser pulse energies, faster scanning speeds, and denser spot placements. This path has weaved a bit over time, because laser photodisruption during femtosecond laser corneal surgery depends on many physical factors, including the parameters that characterize the laser pulse, the laser-scanning method, as well as the details of corneal applanation, including tissue state, depth targeted, shape of cuts, etc. This development path has culminated in the ability of the current VisuMax® laser system to create cuts of sufficient quality that stromal lenticules with curved surfaces can be created and removed to effect a refractive change in the cornea.

In considering the SMILE procedure in particular, one can ask several questions about the surface cut quality. Are the cuts good enough to extract the femto-cut stromal tissue? Are the lenticule edges cut with sufficient quality to prevent edges from tearing upon extraction? Is there any difference between the quality of the lamellar (cap) cuts and refractive power (lenticule) cuts? To address these questions, we first sought an appropriate method for the evaluation of cut surface quality.

Resection quality for femtosecond cuts has been variously defined as resection surface smoothness characterized by microscopy, as subjective grading of the ease of manual dissection, or as the absence of tissue bridges, grooves, cavitation marks, striations, or waviness observed in the stromal bed [12]. In the case of refractive intracorneal lens removal procedures with either a flap (FLEX) or through a small incision (SMILE), the quality and/or accuracy of the cut surfaces is important to visual outcomes and potentially to visual recovery and any inflammatory response. The surface quality of corneal lenticules produced by the related FLEX procedure was evaluated using the first commercially VisuMax system, which operated at a 200 kHz repetition rate [4, 12]. Kunert et al. studied the cut quality of lenticules extracted from clinical patients using three different pulse energies (150 nJ, 180 nJ, and 195 nJ) and a single spot density setting (3 μm × 3 μm) (*see also* Chap. 17) [12]. The highest quality resections were associated with the lowest pulse energy (150 nJ). An additional study created refractive lenticules with the FLEX procedure in cadaver eyes [13] using the next-generation 500 kHz VisuMax system with a pulse energy of 130 nJ and a 3 μm × 3 μm spot density. SEM imaging was performed of the exposed cadaveric corneal stromal beds. Surface quality of the stromal beds was improved over the earlier studies, though the authors observed rough patches and features they attributed to cavitation bubbles in the SEM images.

Traditionally, surface quality of femtosecond laser cut corneal tissue has been performed with scanning electron microscopy (SEM). Since SMILE lenticules are quite thin compared to flap or keratoplasty corneal lamellar resections, artifacts, surface morphology, or roughness may be introduced into lenticule samples by the mounting, critical point drying, and conductive coating processes used in SEM sample preparation [4, 12, 13]. We therefore elected instead to use a related electron microscopy technique called environmental SEM (eSEM) [14]. The eSEM imaging technique is performed on hydrated and uncoated biological samples under low-vacuum conditions, eliminating artifacts due to tissue preparation processes [14].

Although the remaining bed and cap surfaces in the cornea are the actual cut surfaces of interest, directly characterizing these cut surfaces is difficult and perhaps not even possible in a patient. eSEM allows for imaging of both lamellar surfaces of the removed tissue sections (lenticules) of the same piece of tissue. We infer that the cut surfaces remaining in the eye of the patient will be mirror images of the discarded lenticule surfaces, which can be imaged. If the lenticule has good-quality cut surfaces, this will be a reflection of corneal tissue surfaces left in the eye. However, there are artifact-inducing processes which may affect the removed corneal lenticule, such as the mechanical trauma of extraction and removal as well as processes that occur during the manipulation of the extracted tissue during imaging. Caution is warranted in interpreting image information from lenticule cut surfaces, and care must be taken to avoid arriving at incorrect conclusions about defects or abnormalities in corneas based on what may be artifacts in lenticule images. Nonetheless, we feel that valuable information may be gained by a microscopic examination of lenticule surfaces.

We therefore used eSEM comparative analysis to examine the surface quality of the cuts associated with the SMILE procedure performed with the 500 kHz version of the VisuMax® [15]. This examination is likely the first in which the cut quality

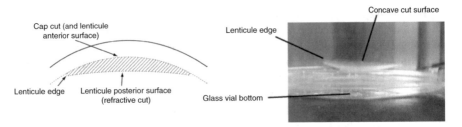

Cap cut (and lenticule anterior surface)

Lenticule edge

Concave cut surface

Lenticule edge   Lenticule posterior surface (refractive cut)

Glass vial bottom

Fig. 16.1 Left graphic depicts geometry of lenticule in a pure-sphere SMILE procedure for reference. Right image is a photographic image of an extracted lenticule, preserved in formalin, prior to electron microscopy. A curvature is readily observed in the lenticule sample, enabling the identification of anterior and posterior surfaces

associated with patients undergoing SMILE for myopia with the 500 kHz and the first in which both lenticule cut surfaces have been examined simultaneously.

A small number of lenticules were extracted from patients undergoing SMILE for spherical myopia at Åarhus University Hospital in Denmark. The VisuMax® laser parameters used for these SMILE patients were repetition rate = 500 kHz, laser energy = 120 nJ, and spot density = 2.5 μm × 2.5 μm. The geometric parameters were lenticule diameter = 6.5 mm, edge thickness = 15 μm, cap diameter = 7.3 mm, and cap thickness = 120 μm. The opening incision width was 60°, and the incision was located at the superior position. Immediately after removal from the eye, lenticules were placed in a light fixative (2 % formalin) and transported to the University of Miami (Coral Gables, FL, USA) for imaging [16]. No additional sample preparation was required. A macroscopic image of a typical lenticule is shown in Fig. 16.1 below.

Samples were imaged using a FEI/Philips XL-30 Field Emission eSEM/SEM microscope [14]. Images were collected from one side of a sample, with the opposite side sample subsequently imaged after removing and reorienting the sample. Images were acquired at three magnifications: 100×, 250×, and 500×. Exemplary eSEM images of five spherical correction lenticules at 100× magnification are shown in Fig. 16.2. The left column of Fig. 16.2 shows views of the convex surfaces and the middle column shows the concave surfaces.

The surfaces of the lenticules were identified as convex and concave by inspection during mounting. Since no orientation marks were made to identify the surfaces

Fig. 16.2 eSEM images of ten lenticule surfaces of five lenticules extracted from SMILE patients. Each row depicts a separate lenticule. Left column is the convex (*top*) surface. Middle column is concave (*bottom*) surface. Spherical correction size for each row is labeled in rightmost column. (**a**) −9.75 D. (**b**) −10.0 D. (**c**) −6.75 D. (**d**) −7.00 D. (**e**) −7.25 D. All images are 250× magnification

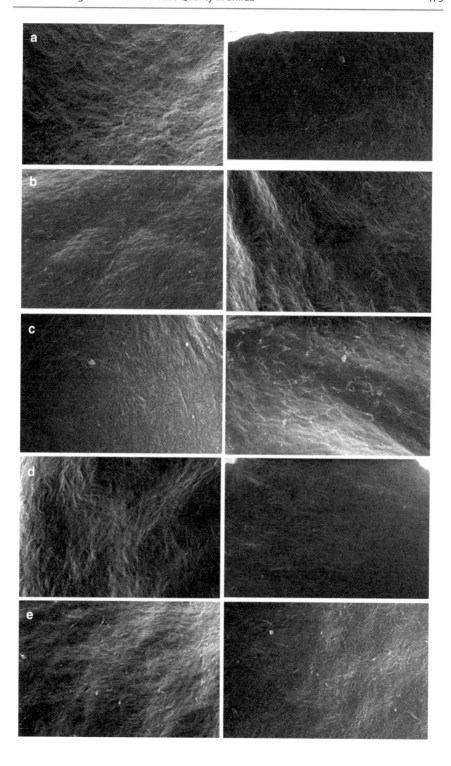

as posterior or anterior, a positive identification of the surface orientation cannot be made. We assume that the corneal lenticules are sufficiently stiff to maintain their natural curvature after removal so that the concave surfaces were likely to correspond to the posterior surfaces. Concave and convex surfaces of the lenticules appear smooth and absent of surface irregularities. Concave and convex surfaces appear equally smooth, with no obvious differences between them. No holes from cavitation bubbles were seen in any of the images. Attachments or tissue bridges appear to be minimal, and the surface morphology appears regular and intact in the highest magnification views.

In SMILE procedures, the quality of the lenticule edge cuts is as important as the general quality of the lamellar-type cut surfaces. Keeping the lenticules intact without tearing or breaks at the edges during lenticule extraction is key to a successful and problem-free procedure. Ideally, the edges of the lenticules would be cut with a clean and well-defined edge. Turning to the images in Fig. 16.3, the lenticule edges are observed at 100× to be well defined and integral for the most part. In Fig. 16.3a, the lenticule sample is folded in such a way that the edge overlays the convex central portion of a lenticule. In contrast, the edge may be jagged in areas where the surgeon has removed or manipulated the lenticule with forceps, as can be seen at one portion of another lenticule edge (Fig. 16.3b). In Fig. 16.3c, the intrinsically good quality of lenticule edge or side cuts can be seen from the concave side. The sample in Fig. 16.3c is mounted on a wire grid, while the other two lenticules in Fig. 16.3 are mounted on flat surfaces.

A direct study of these surfaces by SEM imaging would not be possible in patients, since the cornea itself would have to be processed and imaged. The strength of the imaging technique we have described here is that it allows for an indirect characterization of both lamellar cut surfaces in the patient's eye using a single sample. A weakness is that this characterization depends upon the assumption that the cut surfaces remaining in the patient's cornea are faithfully represented by the quality of the matched lenticule cut surfaces. While a complete validation of this technique would be a comparative study of lenticules from cadaver or animal eyes with the matched corneal beds or corneal cut surfaces, it seems reasonable to infer the cut quality in the cornea by characterizing the cut quality of extracted lenticules.

Our particular technique could benefit from being able to construct a composite image of the entire sample, which we plan to implement using a newer low-vacuum SEM microscope. A validation of the cut quality in donor corneas against the extracted lenticules would strengthen our indirect comparison technique. In addition, adding orientation markings to the lenticule samples would be useful, especially when we examine astigmatic lenticules.

The lower pulse energy and tighter laser spot density SMILE cuts we examined using the 500 kHz VisuMax may be of higher cut quality than those reported for the 200 kHz VisuMax, since lower pulse energies and closer spot placements have often been associated with smoother femtosecond cuts [17]. However, since the SMILE procedure is continuing to be refined, the cut quality may continue to improve. The recent introduction of astigmatic SMILE and FLEX corrections with transition zone features may merit additional investigation to examine whether these additional

Fig. 16.3 Lenticule edge quality. (**a**) Lenticule from the −9.75 D correction previously shown in Fig. 16.2a is folded, with edge overlaying convex surface. (**b**) Edge of a lenticule from a −7 D correction is seen from concave side, with edges damaged, likely by forceps used to surgically manipulate and extract lenticule. (**c**) Lenticule from the −7.25 D correction previously shown in Fig. 16.2e has cleanly cut edges as seen from convex surface. Circular periphery seen in (a) and (b) is the microscope field aperture. All images are 100× magnification

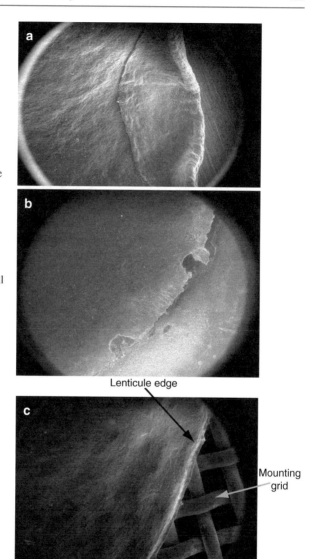

features associated with spherocylindrical lenticules produce results that are consistent with the results described here for sphere-only lenticules. The use of faster scanning times to the period that subject eyes are subject to applanation and suction may also warrant investigation into the effect of next-generation scanning parameters on cut quality.

While examinations of the microscopic quality of the femtosecond laser cut surfaces in the SMILE procedure or in related procedures may produce useful information, it is the macroscopic shape of the lenticule surfaces which is the key factor in achieving desired refractive changes. It should also be recalled that the corneal stroma differs between individual eyes, and the structure of stromal tissue changes with depth within the eye. Interpreting SEM results must be taken with these factors in mind. Ultimately, the clinical results of these procedures is the "gold standard" for evaluation of safety and efficacy, and this characterization method should be viewed as supplemental to clinical evaluations.

At present, we lack direct evidence correlating the smoothness of stromal surfaces and directly clinical outcomes. However, we believe the technique of lenticule surface examination by eSEM provides a useful window into understanding the in vivo surface morphology associated with the corneal shape changes created with the femtosecond lenticule removal procedure. eSEM imaging of lenticules may prove useful in future evaluations of SMILE or related procedures.

Acknowledgements This work was funded by Carl Zeiss Meditec. Imaging was performed at the Center for Advanced Microscopy at the University of Miami in Coral Gables, Florida.

References

1. Juhasz T, Loesel F, Kurtz R, Horvath C, Bille J, Mourou G (1999) Corneal refractive surgery with femtosecond lasers. IEEE J Sel Topics Quant Electron 5(4): 902–910
2. Sarayba MA, Ignacio TS, Binder PS, Tran DB (2007) Comparative study of stromal bed quality by using mechanical, IntraLase femtosecond laser 15- and 30-kHz microkeratomes. Cornea 26:446–451
3. Sarayba MA, Ignacio TS, Tran DB, Binder PS (2007) A 60 kHz IntraLase femtosecond laser creates a smoother LASIK stromal bed surface compared to a Zyoptix XP mechanical microkeratome in human donor eyes. J Refract Surg 23:331–337
4. Kunert KS, Blum M, Duncker GI, Sietmann R, Heichel J (2011) Surface quality of human corneal lenticules after femtosecond laser surgery for myopia comparing different laser parameters. Graefes Arch Clin Exp Ophthalmol 249:1417–1424
5. Sarayba MA, Maguen E, Salz J, Rabinowitz Y, Ignacio TS (2007) Femtosecond laser keratome creation of partial thickness donor corneal buttons for lamellar keratoplasty. J Refract Surg 23:58–65
6. Terry MA, Ousley PJ, Will B (2005) A practical femtosecond laser procedure for DLEK endothelial transplantation: cadaver eye histology and topography. Cornea 24:453–459
7. Vinciguerra P, Azzolini M, Radice P, Sborgia M, De Molfetta V (1998) A method for examining surface and interface irregularities after photorefractive keratectomy and laser in situ keratomileusis: predictor of optical and functional outcomes. J Refract Surg 14:S204–S206
8. Stonecipher KG, Dishler JG, Ignacio TS, Binder PS (2006) Transient light sensitivity after femtosecond laser flap creation: clinical findings and management. J Cataract Refract Surg 32:91–94
9. Niemz M, Hoppeler T, Juhasz T, Bille J (1993) Intrastromal ablations for refractive corneal surgery using picosecond infrared laser pulses. Lasers Light Ophthalmol 5:149–155
10. Holzer M (2009) Update on intraCOR. J Cataract Refract Surg 44–45
11. Seyeddain O, Bachernegg A, Riha W, Rückl T, Reitsamer H, Grabner G, Dexl A (2013) Femtosecond laser–assisted small-aperture corneal inlay implantation for corneal compensation of presbyopia: two-year follow-up. J Cataract Refract Surg 39(2):234–241
12. Heichel J, Blum M, Duncker GI, Sietmann R, Kunert KS (2011) Surface quality of porcine corneal lenticules after femtosecond lenticule extraction. Ophthalmic Res 46(2):107–112
13. Ang M, Chaurasia SS, Angunawela RI et al (2012) Femtosecond lenticule extraction (FLEx): clinical results, interface evaluation, and intraocular pressure variation. Invest Ophthalmol Vis Sci 53:1414–1421

14. Kirk SE, Skepper JN, Donald AM (2009) Application of environmental scanning electron microscopy to determine biological surface structure. J Microsc 233:205–224
15. Ziebarth N, Lorenzo M, Chow J, Cabot F, Spooner G, Dishler J, Hjortdal J, Yoo S (2014) Surface quality of human corneal lenticules after SMILE assessed using environmental scanning electron microscopy. J Refract Surg 30(6):388–393
16. Human Subjects Research Office, University of Miami, Miami, Florida USA 33136. "Assessment of Cut Quality of Corneal Lenticules", study #20120444.
17. Faktorovich E (2009) Femtodynamics: a guide to laser settings and procedure techniques to optimize outcomes with femtosecond lasers. SLACK, Thorofare, pp 20–22. ISBN 13 978-1-55642-862-3

Collagen Characteristics and Refractive Outcomes

17

Kathleen S. Kunert, Marcus Blum, Thabo Lapp,
and Claudia Auw-Hädrich

Content

High satisfaction after refractive surgery fundamentally depends on the long-term refractive stability. Several factors have an influence on postoperative refractive results, i.e. long-term stability of preoperative refraction, preoperative difference between subjective and objective refractive measurements. Individual tissue characteristics might have an influence on postoperative results as well. However, there are no options up to now to evaluate tissue parameters preoperatively.

Attempted and achieved corrections have already been analysed in FLEx and SMILE. The femtosecond lenticule extraction procedure now offers the unique opportunity of obtaining healthy human corneal tissue for morphological analysis.

To further evaluate and thereby improve the visual outcome after the FLEx procedure, we analysed the correlation between the following electron microscopical findings of FLEx lenticules and pre-, intra- and postoperative parameters: The correlation between *clinical* parameters, (1) preoperative contact lens (CL) type and time of daily use, (2) intraoperative separability of the lenticules, (3) postoperative accuracy of refraction, (4) regression/deviation from target refraction and (5) patient's age and *morphological* parameters, (1) collagen fibre diameter, (2) area of extracellular matrix substance between the collagen fibres, (3) collagen fibre

K.S. Kunert (✉) • M. Blum
Department of Ophthalmology, HELIOS Klinikum Erfurt, Erfurt, Germany
e-mail: kathleen.kunert@helios-kliniken.de; marcus.blum@helios-kliniken.de

T. Lapp • C. Auw-Hädrich
University Eye Centre Freiburg, Albert-Ludwigs-University, Freiburg im Breisgau, Germany
e-mail: thabo.lapp@uniklinik-freiburg.de; claudia.auw-haedrich@uniklinik-freiburg.de

© Springer International Publishing Switzerland 2015
W. Sekundo (ed.), *Small Incision Lenticule Extraction (SMILE):
Principles, Techniques, Complication Management, and Future Concepts*,
DOI 10.1007/978-3-319-18530-9_17

179

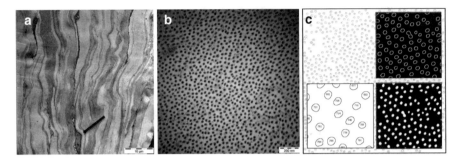

Fig. 17.1 Electron microscopy and ImageJ analysis – overview pictures (**a**, bar=50 µm) were taken to select areas with cross cut collagen fibres. A single keratocyte can be detected in this overview (*arrow*). Higher-resolution pictures were used for analysis (**b**, bar=200 nm). Using ImageJ single collagen fibres were circled (*upper right panel*), filled (*lower right panel*) and counted (background picture and higher resolution down left) (With kind permission from Klinische Monatsblätter für Augenheilkunde.)

density and (4) homogeneity of the collagen fibres of FLEx lenticules, was analysed. Finally we looked for a correlation between visual recovery, age and different morphological parameters.

Thirty lenticules (of 18 myopic and 12 hyperopic eyes) of 22 patients were included. Ultra-thin cuts (78 nm) of embedded lenticules were prepared for transmission electron microscopy (TEM). TEM samples were analysed using ImageJ analysis (version 1.45s, NIH, USA); see Fig. 17.1.

The main findings of the study are as follows:

(a) Intraoperative lenticule dissection difficulties

   Nine out of the 30 lenticules were difficult to dissect. The difficulty of lenticule dissection was determined on the basis of surgical video analysis prior to statistical analysis.

   A thicker collagen fibre diameter involves a potential risk for increased intraoperative lenticule adhesiveness ($p=0.056$). Vice versa a higher fibre distance and a lower fibre density, respectively, significantly reduce the risk of intraoperative difficulty in dissecting a lenticule ($p=0.036$); see Fig. 17.2. Furthermore, a higher coefficient of variation (CV) of fibre density also seems to reduce the risk for lenticule adhesiveness ($p=0.033$).

   The odds ratio for a difficult lenticule dissection in patients who wore contact lenses (CL) was 0.06 in comparison with non-CL users ($p=0.03$). An odds ratio of 0.06 means that the risk of a complicated surgery (intraoperative lenticule adhesiveness) is significantly reduced to 6 % by long-time CL wear. Vice versa in older patients, the risk for intraoperative complications is annually increased to 11 % ($p=0.09$).

(b) Regression

   The deviation (i.e. the difference of the spherical equivalent 12 months after surgery minus the spherical equivalent 6 months post-surgery) showed

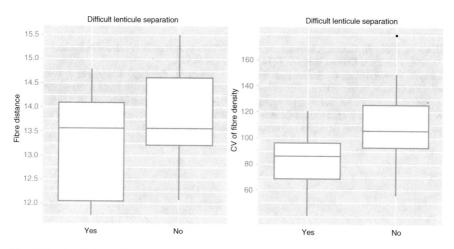

Fig. 17.2 Correlation of intraoperative lenticule separability and fibre distance and its coefficient of variation, respectively. The correlation of intraoperative difficult lenticule separability and collagen fibre distance (**a**) and coefficient of variation (*CV*) of fibre density (**b**) showed significant findings

significant correlation to the CV of fibre distance ($p=0.02$); thus, higher grades of inhomogeneity of the fibre distance seem to be associated with an increased risk of postoperative myopic regression.

Moreover, regression was significantly associated ($p=0.05$) with the time of preoperative contact lens use: a longer period of contact lens use seems to increase the risk of postoperative regression towards myopia.

From this study we can summarise that smaller fibre diameters, resulting in a larger distance, respectively a lower fibre density as well as a higher fibre inhomogeneity reduce the difficulty of intraoperative flap and lenticule separation. Regarding the preoperative clinical parameters, a longer preoperative period of contact lens use had protective effects on the surgical procedure, whilst an advanced age tended to constitute a risk factor for adhesiveness of the lenticule.

A high coefficient of variation of fibre spacing and a high cumulative contact lens wearing time seem to increase the risk of regression towards myopia. Low fibre density and thus higher fibre distances, longer contact lens wearing time and higher age at the time of surgery tend to increase the risk of poorer visual outcome.

Some of these findings could possibly be taken into consideration in decision-making for refractive surgery and be used as prognostic parameters for postoperative visual recovery and development of refraction. Nevertheless, the findings of this study need to be examined in a larger cohort to test their clinical validity and applicability. One major drawback is that the morphological parameters cannot be evaluated in vivo so far. Clinical implication of the data is therefore limited and can only be used for patients who already had their surgery. However, the impact of prolonged contact lens wear should be considered and discussed with the patient *before* surgery.

Related Literature

Blum M, Flach A, Kunert KS, Sekundo W (2014) Five-year results of refractive lenticule extraction. J Cataract Refract Surg 40(9):1425–1429

Lapp T, Auw-Hädrich C, Sadler F, Böhringer D, Blum M, Reinhard T, Heichel J, Kunert KS (2014) Morphological analysis of corneal refractive lenticules--is there a correlation with refractive results? Klin Monbl Augenheilkd 231(7):690–696. Epub 2014 Jul 18. German

Mohamed-Noriega K et al (2011) Cornea lenticule viability and structural integrity after refractive lenticule extraction (ReLEx) and cryopreservation. Mol Vis 17:3437–3449

Part IV
Future Concepts

SMILE for Correction of Very High Myopia (Higher than −10 D)

18

Osama Ibrahim, Moones Abdalla, Amro Saeed, Kitty Mohammed, and Ibrahim Ahmed

Content

In spite of the presence of several treatment modalities for correcting myopias higher than −10 D, the surgical treatment is still considered one of the biggest challenges a refractive surgeon can face to this day. Such modalities comprise refractive lens exchange (RLE), phakic IOL (pIOL), LASIK, and surface ablation [1].

RLE and phakic IOLs, being intraocular procedures, carry the risks of endophthalmitis, surgically induced astigmatism, and loss of corneal endothelial cells. RLE is additionally associated with the risk of retinal detachment and generally is not considered in pre-presbyopic patients with myopia who can still accommodate, whereas phakic IOLs are associated with pupillary block glaucoma, pigment dispersion syndrome and cataract formation for the ICL, and progressive endothelial cell loss for anterior chamber pIOLs. Also biometry and surgical implantation of phakic IOLs require special techniques and the long-term outcomes of several types of phakic IOLs are unknown [1].

LASIK and PRK with MMC are no longer considered reasonable options for the treatment of myopias over −10 D as they are less predictable than treatments for lower levels of myopia. Haze has been reported to be a significant long-term problem in eyes with high myopia treated with PRK [2]. Studies that evaluated the long-term outcomes of PRK in high myopes have shown that regression was observed despite single or double application of MMC [3].

O. Ibrahim (✉) • M. Abdalla • A. Saeed • K. Mohammed • I. Ahmed
Roayah Vision Correction Center, Alexandria University, Alexandria, Egypt
e-mail: ibrosama@gmail.com

© Springer International Publishing Switzerland 2015
W. Sckundo (cd.), *Small Incision Lenticule Extraction (SMILE): Principles, Techniques, Complication Management, and Future Concepts*,
DOI 10.1007/978-3-319-18530-9_18

As described in Chap. 13 by Reinstein et al., it is reasonable to assume that SMILE will leave the cornea with greater postoperative tensile strength than LASIK or PRK for any given refractive correction, provided the strongest anterior stroma remains uncut. This is of particular importance for very high myopic treatments, because of the large amount of corneal tissue to be removed which predisposes patients to the risk of corneal ectasia. In SMILE, the high accuracy of cap thickness described in the literature provides evidence for biomechanical stability within the cap as well as the stroma in the residual bed. As for the functional optical zone in SMILE (i.e., size of the treated area that has achieved good optical performance [4]), it was observed that the topographic flattening after surgery was wider than the flattening achieved by the same optical zone when performed with excimer ablation.

Since the time required to correct a −14 D is equal to that required to correct a −1 D using SMILE (provided that both have the same optical zone and cap size), factors influencing photoablative procedures' precision such as room humidity, corneal hydration, parallax error, laser fluency, and above all the excessive heat produced are all eliminated.

Other considerations where SMILE results compared favorably to LASIK included corneal sensation and ocular surface condition, higher-order aberration induction, wound healing and inflammatory responses responsible for postoperative proliferation, and possible regression.

Based on all the considerations mentioned above, we investigated a possible use of SMILE technique for patients with myopias higher than −10 D as our research software allows correction of up to −14 D. Our study included 382 eyes treated for a mean error of −12.48 ± 1.76 D (range: −10.0 to −14.0 D) combined with mean astigmatism −1.26 ± 1.04 D (up to −4.0 D). The mean CDVA was 0.67 ± 0.94 (range: 0.5–1.0). At 6 months after surgery, 365 eyes had mean refractive error −1.28 ± 1.76 (range: +0.75 to −3.25 D) and mean postoperative astigmatism −0.83 ± 1.04 D (up to −1.75 D). The mean CDVA reached 0.74 ± 0.4 (range: 0.5–1.0) at 6 months follow-up. At 1 year, 280 eyes had a mean error of −1.83 ± 1.33 D (range: +0.5 to −4.25 D), mean astigmatism of −0.76 ± 1.04 D (up to −2.0 D) and CDVA 0.79 ± 0.4 (range: 0.5–1.0). By the end of the follow-up period, about 94 % of patients had unchanged CDVA or gained 1 or more lines, 6 % lost 1 line of CDVA, and 1 % lost 2 lines along the follow-up period. We had no significant regression and not a single case of ectasia. Figures 18.1 and 18.2 show representative pre- and postoperative Pentacam® images.

This procedure was performed on corneas with minimum CCT of not less than 500 μm, ensuring that at least 250 μm of residual stromal bed is left and at least 100 μm cap thickness. The lenticule diameter (i.e., optical zone) was adjusted according to the scotopic pupil diameter and the residual stroma. Therefore, there should be a balance between the residual stromal bed thickness, pupil diameter, and lenticule diameter.

As the machine's settings have the tendency of undercorrection, we adjusted our nomogram to add about 5–15 % of the manifest refraction according to the patients' age. However, some patients were intentionally undercorrected due to age considerations, high numerical sum of sphere and cylinder (higher than 14), or insufficient

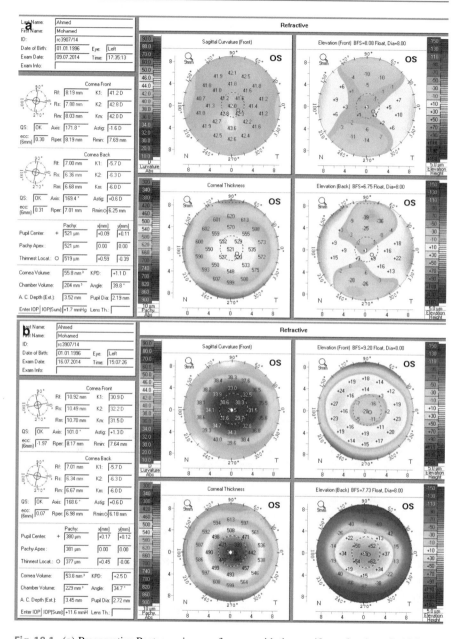

Fig. 18.1 (**a**) Preoperative Pentacam image of an eye with the manifest refraction of −12.0 −1.0 @ 165°. (**b**) Same eye 1 week postoperatively. The manifest refraction (MR) is +0.25 −0.5 @ 120°. There is a distinct elevation of the posterior corneal surface. (**c**) After 3 months both the refraction and the topography remain unchanged: +0.25 +0.25 @ 100°

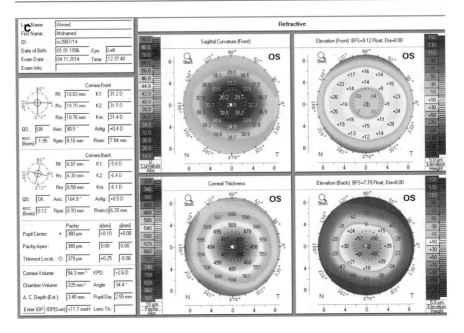

Fig. 18.1 (continued)

corneal thickness. In some cases we had to compromise the astigmatism correction in order to salvage the correction of very high spheres.

In the light of our current results, we believe that higher errors up to −16 D or even up to −18 D might be corrected with the same safety and predictability. Because of the novel nature of high correction, we kept the residual stroma over 250 μm similarly to Lasik. However, as described in Chap. 13, the residual stroma thickness is a term used in flap-based surgery like Lasik or FLEx. The total corneal thickness is more applicable for SMILE surgery (see Chap. 13). Moreover, thicker caps and thinner posterior stroma might be even more advantageous than settings used in current investigation. As SMILE is still an evolving procedure, further experimental investigations of post-SMILE biomechanics and optics will shed more light and help to define the boundaries of corneal refractive correction.

Importantly, whenever enhancement was required, PRK with 0.02 % MMC for 20 s was our choice in order not to lose the advantages rendered by the SMILE technique.

Finally, SMILE is a reversible procedure. The lenticule removed may be stored and replaced into the cornea at a later time (see Chap. 20). This adds the advantage of potentially reversing the refractive procedure when the patient develops presbyopia. Reimplantation of the lenticule may also allow the treatment of ectasia and the reversal of myopia [5].

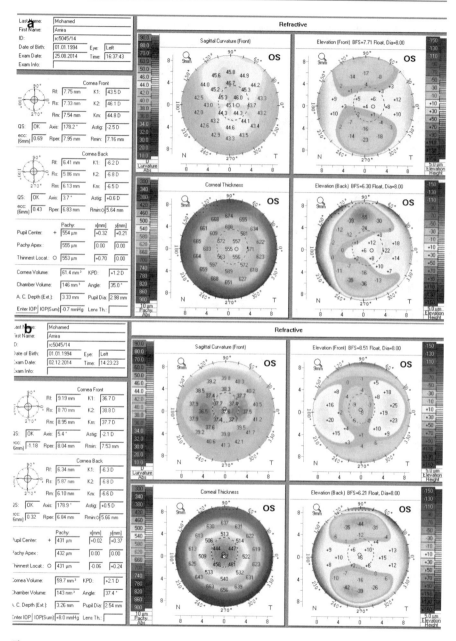

Fig. 18.2 (**a**) Another example of high myopia combined with astigmatism. MR =−14.0 −2.0 @ 10°. (**b**) Three months after surgery with primary under-correction for sphere and cylinder the MR is −2.0 −1.25 @ 30°. The posterior float is virtually unchanged. (**c**) Anterior curvature difference map (right column) between pre-op (left column) and 3 months post-op (middle column). Also note that despite very high correction the residual corneal power is well above 37 D

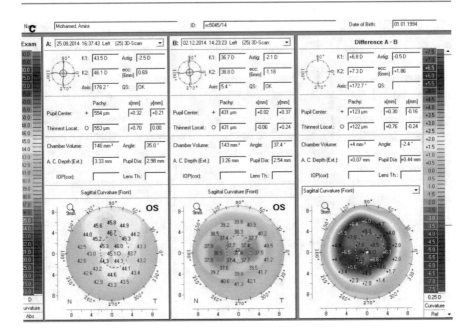

Fig. 18.2 (continued)

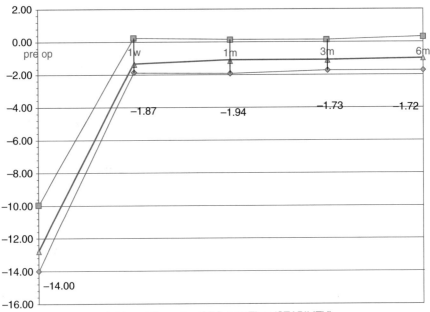

Achieved Correction SEQ over Time 'STABILITY'

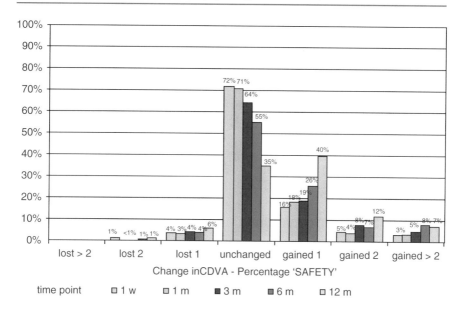

References

1. Barsam A (2012) Surgical treatment of high myopia. Cataract and refractive surgery today: peer review. Available from: http://crstoday.com/2012/06/surgical-treatment-of-high-myopia/. Accessed 19 Oct 2014
2. Lindstrom RL, Sher NA, Barak M et al (1992) Excimer laser photorefractive keratectomy in high myopia: a multicentre study. Trans Am Ophthalmol Soc 90:277–296; discussion 296–301
3. Fazel F, Naderibeni A, Eslami F, Ghatrehsamani H (2008) Results of photorefractive keratectomy with mitomycin C for high myopia after 4 years. JRMS 13:80–87
4. Tabernero J, Klyce SD, Sarver EJ, Artal P (2007) Functional optical zone of the cornea. Invest Ophthalmol Vis Sci 48(3):1053–1060
5. Ang M, Tan D, Mehta JS (2012) Small incision lenticule extraction (SMILE) versus laser in-situ keratomileusis (LASIK): study protocol for a randomised, non- inferiority trial. Trial 13:75

Hyperopic Correction by ReLEx®

19

Walter Sekundo, Dan Z. Reinstein, Kishore Pradhan, and Marcus Blum

Contents

19.1   Hyperopic Correction by ReLEx® FLEx

Despite an increasing popularity of the ReLEx® procedure, it still has some drawbacks. One of them is the absence of software for the current VisuMax® laser to treat hyperopia. Indeed, the idea of "all-in-one surgery" can only become a true femtosecond-laser-alone procedure, if all refractive errors can be treated without excimer laser.

W. Sekundo (✉)
Department of Ophthalmology, Philipps University of Marburg and Universitätsklinikum Giessen & Marburg GmbH, Marburg, Germany
e-mail: sekundo@med.uni-marburg.de

D.Z. Reinstein
London Vision Clinic, 138 Harley Street, London, UK

Columbia University Medical Center, New York, NY, USA

K. Pradhan
Tilganga Institute of Ophthalmology, Kathmandu, Nepal

M. Blum
Department of Ophthalmology, HELIOS- Hospital Erfurt, Erfurt, Germany

© Springer International Publishing Switzerland 2015
W. Sekundo (ed.), *Small Incision Lenticule Extraction (SMILE):*
Principles, Techniques, Complication Management, and Future Concepts,
DOI 10.1007/978-3-319-18530-9_19

19.1.1 The First Study

Our group published the first paper on this topic in 2013 [1]. In this study, we performed FLEx in 47 hyperopic eyes of 26 patients utilizing the 200 kHz VisuMax® femtosecond laser system. Forty-two out of 47 hyperopic eyes of the treatment group completed the final 9 months follow-up. The patients' mean age was 42.3 (±9.0) years. Their preoperative mean spherical equivalent (SE) was +2.80 ± 1.3 D (range +1.25 to +4.0 D). The authors (W.S., M.B.) performed all surgeries. Intended flap thickness was 120 μm. Because of the longer treatment time with the 200 kHz laser as compared to today's 500 kHz laser, we used the S "contact glass" in the vast majority of treated eyes. Thus, the flap diameter was chosen between 7.0 and 8.5 mm depending on the lenticule diameter. In all cases, a superior hinge, 50° in chord length, was left. The lenticule diameter varied between 6.2 and 7.6 mm according to patient's mesopic pupil diameter and white-to-white distance. The lenticule's minimal thickness varied between 20 and 25 μm. In this first study, we used a pseudo-transition zone created by an oblique (slope-like) angle of the lenticule edge. Nine months post-operatively, 64 % of eyes treated were within ±1.00 D and 38 % of eyes within ±0.50 D of intended correction. One eye out of 47 (2.1 %) lost more than two Snellen lines, but none of the eyes had UCVA less than

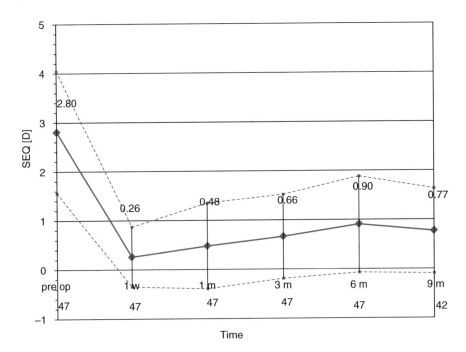

Fig. 19.1 Stability of refractive outcome over the 9-month follow-up period in the initial hyperopic study (Reprinted from Blum et al. [1])

20/40. While we could show that hyperopic treatment was feasible and that good centration was not an issue, the rate of refractive regression (Fig. 19.1) was unacceptable in comparison to modern excimer laser correction of low to moderate hyperopia [2]. Thus, several patients have received excimer laser enhancement. Moreover, we had one serious complication with a lenticule remnant in the centre of the optical zone, due to a buttonhole through the lenticule, leading to a "central island" appearance.

19.1.2 The Second (Ongoing) Hyperopic FLEx Study

An improved lenticule shape was developed (Fig. 19.2) that had identical optical properties within the optical zone as in the original study, but with a number of differences mainly relating to the creation of a dedicated transition zone. The key features of the larger transition zone were based on the positive long-term experience with hyperopic ablation profiles of the MEL 80 excimer laser [2, 3]. The transition zone was selected for each case individually, according to the corneal curvature, lenticule optical zone diameter, and the dioptric power of treatment (Fig. 19.2).

However, the total extent of the optical zone and transition zone is limited by the size of the VisuMax® contact glass being used, as the contact glass is applied to the cornea for suction. Therefore, in order to maximize the total lenticule diameter, we used a medium (M)-size contact glass in all cases rather than a small (S)-size contact glass as in the majority of eyes in the previous study (similarly to myopic treatments). In order to obtain treatment zones as large as possible, the clearance between the edge of the lenticule and the edge of the flap was reduced

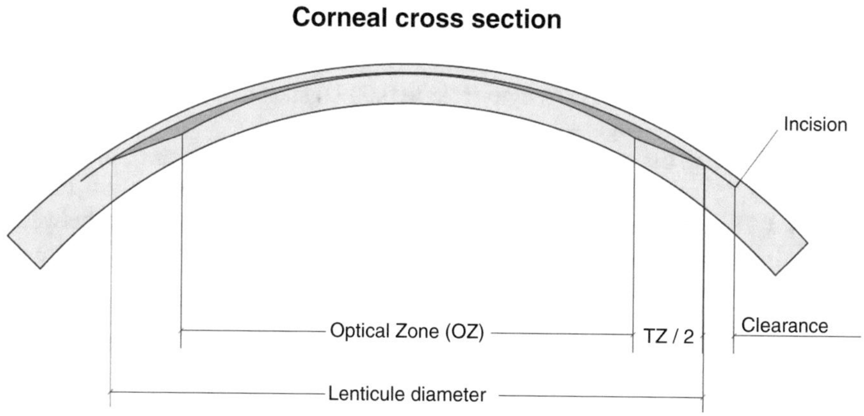

Corneal cross section

Fig. 19.2 Diagram of the improved lenticule shape used in the present study. Note a large transition zone and the minimal lenticule thickness at the edge and in the centre

to as low as 0.5 mm, compared to the 1 mm clearance that was used in the first study. When planning the lenticule and flap dimensions, the corneal diameter was also considered; as the treatments were centred on the corneal vertex, the flap diameter was confirmed to be within the diameter of the cornea in cases with an angle kappa, where the centre of the treatment would not be aligned with the centre of the cornea.

The other change between the two studies was that the pulse frequency of the VisuMax® had been increased from 200 to 500 kHz. This increase in pulse frequency meant that the new lenticule shape (with increased optical zone, transition zone, and flap diameters) could be performed without increasing the total treatment time and therefore did not affect safety in relation to the risk of suction loss.

Because of the above-mentioned complication in the first study, where one eye developed a central buttonhole in the lenticule [1], we paid a lot of attention to the question of the central minimum lenticule thickness. After extensive ex vivo experiments with pig eyes and human corneas not eligible for corneal transplantation, this value was set at 25 μm in all eyes without any exception, rather than sometimes using 20 μm in the first study.

The Ethics Committees recommended that the study be divided into a pilot study with ten eyes (initial spherical cohort) to be followed by a larger study of 40 eyes (second, spherocylindrical cohort) only after the 9-month data had been reported for the first treatment group. Therefore, only the results of the nine eyes of five patients of the pilot study are available at present (N.B. one patient was emmetropic in one eye).

Patients' average age at the time of surgery was 55.5 (range: 46–63) years. One patient (two eyes) was male and the other four patients were female. The mean preoperative manifest spherical equivalent refraction (SE) was $+1.82 \pm 0.56$ D (range: $+1.25$ to $+2.75$ D) with mean preoperative sphere of $+1.89 \pm 0.59$ D (range: $+1.25$ to $+3.00$ D) and mean astigmatism of -0.14 ± 0.18 D (range: 0 to -0.50 D). As all patients were of presbyopic age, an overcorrection was intended in all cases: mean target SE was -0.86 ± 0.41D (range -1.25 to 0.00 D) such that mean attempted SE was $+2.69 \pm 0.39$ D (range: $+2.25$ to $+3.50$ D).

The mean flap diameter was 8.46 ± 0.09 mm (range: 8.4–8.6 mm), the optical zone was 5.75 mm for all eyes, and the mean transition zone was 2.02 ± 0.14 mm (range: 1.78–2.29 mm). The femtosecond laser energy was adjusted between 180 and 160 nJ during the study with a fixed laser spot and track distance of 4.5 μm.

At 1 month, 3 months, 6 months, and 9 months, 33 %, 67 %, 22 %, and 22 % of eyes were within 0.50 D of intended correction, and 78 % of eyes were within 1.00 D of target refraction. The analysis of attempted versus achieved refraction over time shows a regression between month 3 and month 9 of approximately 0.50 D in all but two eyes which were overcorrected. There were neither decentrations nor any other adverse effects (Fig. 19.3). Despite a mean refractive undercorrection of approximately 0.17 D, all patients were happy with the achieved results, simply because we purposely aimed at low myopia and, in this way, managed to bring all eyes into a comfortable zone for the presbyopic age (Fig. 19.4). As planned, larger cohorts will be treated in 2015.

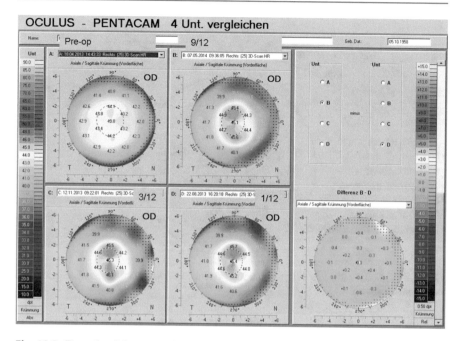

Fig. 19.3 Example of the pre- and post-op topography with steepened and well-centred central cornea (**a**: pre-op, **b**: 9 months, **c**: 3 months, **d**: 6 months after surgery). Also note that the differential map (**b–d**) shows minute changes only while the optical zone measures 6 mm on Pentacam's scale

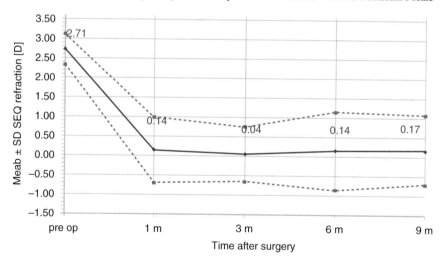

Fig. 19.4 Stability of the manifest refraction shown as change in spherical equivalent over time

19.2 Hyperopic Correction by ReLEx SMILE: The Ongoing Study

Pradhan and Reinstein presented the first results of hyperopic SMILE using two 2 mm incisions at the APAC Meeting 2014. They designed a multiphase study starting with four blind eyes, followed by six densely amblyopic eyes and ten mildly

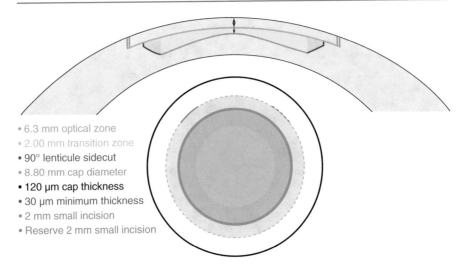

Fig. 19.5 Schematic diagram of hyperopic SMILE lenticule geometry as being used in Pradhan and Reinstein's study

amblyopic eyes. After this, up to 200 normal eyes are planned to be treated. The lenticule shape was partially reminiscent to the one mentioned above, but the optical zone of 6.3 mm was much larger, a transition zone of 2 mm was used for all eyes, and the minimal thickness was set to 30 μm (Fig. 19.5).

Study inclusion criteria were a maximum intended sphere up to +7.00 D with astigmatism up to 6.00 D, age ≥21 years, CDVA 20/100 or worse. Retinoscopic refraction and Atlas topography were obtained before and 1 month after surgery. Twenty eyes were included, and 1-month data were available in 11 eyes at the time of writing. MEL80 corneal vertex-centred LASIK eyes matched for sphere and cylinder (±0.50 D) were randomly mined from our database to make two control groups: optical zone 6.50 or 7.00 mm (both with a 2 mm transition zone diameter). Mean SEQ was +4.68 ± 1.30 D (range: +3.00 to +6.42 D). Mean refractive astigmatism was 1.09 ± 0.65 D (range: 0.50–2.75 D).

Mean post-op SEQ was +0.10 ± 0.91 D (range: −1.16 to +1.50 D) with 27 % of eyes within ±0.50 D and 82 % within ±1.00 D of the target SEQ (N.B. these were retinoscopy refractions in blind or densely amblyopic eyes). Mean spherical aberration change was −0.49 μm in the 6.3 mm SMILE group, which was found to be equivalent to the 7 mm LASIK group (−0.47 μm, $p = 0.916$), but less than the 6.5 mm LASIK group (−0.79 μm, $p = 0.002$).

Optical zone centration was analysed using the difference map of the Atlas tangential curvature to measure the distance between the centre of the optical zone and the corneal vertex (the intended treatment centre). Mean optical zone offset was equal for all groups ($p > 0.73$), being 0.30 ± 0.18 mm in the 6.3 mm SMILE group, 0.34 ± 0.26 mm in the 7 mm LASIK group, and 0.29 ± 0.15 mm in the 6.5 mm LASIK group. This demonstrated that the centration in SMILE was equivalent to LASIK despite the fact that SMILE does not use an eye tracker.

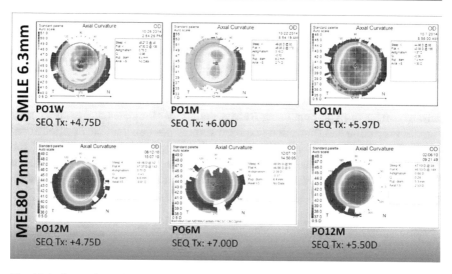

Fig. 19.6 Comparison of achieved optical zones with 6.3 mm lenticule diameter and 7 mm ablation zone showing a slight superiority of SMILE-treated eyes

Mean achieved optical zone diameter was 5.55 ± 0.35 mm in the 6.3 mm SMILE group, which was found to be larger than the 6.5 mm LASIK group (4.65 ± 0.18 mm, $p < 0.001$) and the 7 mm LASIK group (4.93 ± 0.32 mm, $p < 0.001$). Figure 19.6 shows three example postoperative topographies from this hyperopic SMILE population alongside the topography of a matched LASIK case. These examples visually demonstrate the encouraging optical zone diameter and centration results for SMILE.

In summary, optical zone centration was equivalent between vertex-centred hyperopic SMILE and LASIK. Less spherical aberration was induced by 6.3 mm SMILE than 6.5 mm LASIK and was equivalent to 7 mm LASIK. Achieved topographic optical zone diameter was larger for 6.3 mm SMILE than 6.5 and 7 mm LASIK. Refraction change by retinoscopy appeared relatively accurate although longer-term sighted eye studies will be required to refine nomograms and balance these with observed regression.

19.3 Discussion

While the first study showed a feasibility of hyperopic correction by femtosecond laser alone, the current ongoing studies deliver results comparable to the current state-of-the-art excimer laser correction. Three major issues appear to be satisfactorily answered by these investigations:

1. The patient's "self centration" (see also Chap. 14) appears to work well in hyperopic eyes, where the centration issue is more crucial compared to myopic treatments.

2. The results achieved are reasonably stable and can be used for nomogram development.
3. Lenticule parameters as described above appear to satisfy the requirements to safely dissect and remove a lenticule.

Apart from the advantages known from myopic SMILE (see Chaps. 2, 3 and 13), treatment of hyperopia using ReLEx definitely eliminates any excimer laser fluence projection and truncation (exposed stromal bed smaller than ablation zone) errors. The authors are therefore convinced that hyperopic SMILE will enrich the refractive correction choice in the foreseeable future. We will also see the limits of hyperopic corneal surgery based on tissue extraction as opposed to tissue addition (see Chap. 20).

References

1. Blum M, Kunert KS, Voßmerbäumer U, Sekundo W (2013) Femtosecond-lentikel-extraction (ReLEX) corrections for hyperopia – first results. Graefes Arch Clin Exp Ophthalmol 251:349–355
2. Reinstein DZ, Couch DG, Archer TJ (2009) LASIK for hyperopic astigmatism and presbyopia using micro-monovision with the Carl Zeiss Meditec MEL80 platform. J Refract Surg 25(1):37–58
3. Reinstein DZ, Archer TJ, Gobbe M, Silverman RH, Coleman DJ (2010) Epithelial thickness after hyperopic LASIK: three-dimensional display with Artemis very high-frequency digital ultrasound. J Refract Surg 26:555–564

Concept of Reversible Corneal Refractive Surgery (Lenticule Reimplantation)

20

Debbie Tan and Jodhbir S. Mehta

Contents

20.1 Introduction

Refractive lenticule extraction (ReLEx) is a new corneal refractive procedure in which the femtosecond (FS) laser cuts an intrastromal lenticule corresponding to the patients' refractive correction, without the use of microkeratome or excimer laser [1]. The lenticule is then removed through a surface incision of varying size

D. Tan
Cornea and External Disease and Refractive Service, Singapore Eye Research Institute, Singapore, Singapore
Singapore National Eye Centre, Singapore, Singapore
e-mail: jodmehta@gmail.com

J.S. Mehta (✉)
Cornea and External Disease and Refractive Service, Singapore Eye Research Institute, Singapore, Singapore
Singapore National Eye Centre, Singapore, Singapore
Department of Clinical Sciences, Duke-NUS Graduate Medical School, Singapore, Singapore

© Springer International Publishing Switzerland 2015
W. Sekundo (ed.), *Small Incision Lenticule Extraction (SMILE):*
Principles, Techniques, Complication Management, and Future Concepts,
DOI 10.1007/978-3-319-18530-9_20

depending on whether the femtosecond lenticule extraction (FLEx) [2] or small incision lenticule extraction (SMILE) [3, 4] procedure is being performed.

A significant advantage of the SMILE form of ReLEx surgery is the flapless nature of the procedure whereby the lenticule is extracted through a small pocket incision, obviating most flap-related complications. Another potential advantage of ReLEx is that it could be a reversible refractive procedure: The removal of the fully intact refractive intrastromal lenticule in situ allows the possibility of reimplantation. However, to achieve this, the keratocyte viability and overall collagen structural integrity of the extracted stroma lenticule must be maintained. The concept of preserving this lenticule for either subsequent reimplantation into the same patient or as allograft donor tissue in other patients has formed the basis of the first reversible laser refractive procedure.

Previous studies have long shown that corneal tissue can be stored using cryopreservation [5–7], although the process of freezing and thawing has also been shown to damage corneal endothelium and stroma [7–9]. However, it is now possible to cryopreserve the extracted lenticule and reimplant it back into the donor cornea as a method of autologous stromal volume restoration. Recent studies have shown that the stromal lenticule can be preserved to remain viable after cryopreservation and thawing [10]. The intrastromal keratocytes remained viable, undifferentiated, and expressed markers typical of keratocytes from fresh tissue [10].

20.2 Cryopreservation Technique

The developed cryopreservation technique for lenticules was as follows [10, 11]: Extracted lenticules were washed in a phosphate-buffered saline (PBS) buffered antibiotic/antimycotic solution and then transferred into a cryovial and resuspended in 500 µl medium containing 10 % fetal bovine serum (FBS). A stock freezing solution containing 10 % FBS and 20 % dimethyl sulfoxide (DMSO; Sigma, St. Louis, MO), a nontoxic cryoprotectant, was added making up a final volume of 1 ml freezing solution containing 10 % FBS and 10 % DMSO. This helped to prevent intralenticular cell damage during freezing in liquid nitrogen [12]. Freezing of the cryovial containing the stromal lenticule was carried out at a controlled cooling rate within a cryo-container ("Mr. Frosty"; Thermo Fisher Scientific, Roskilde, Denmark) in a −80°C freezer overnight and transferred into liquid nitrogen the following day for long-term storage (1 month). This approach has been shown to reduce the damage caused by intracellular ice formation [11]. After 1 month, the vial with the frozen stromal lenticule was rapidly thawed in a water bath at 37°C and rinsed twice in a PBS solution to remove cryoprotectant agents.

20.3 Ultrastructural Analysis

There was a similar pattern of apoptotic and quiescent keratocytes observed in the fresh and cryopreserved lenticules by transmission electron microscopy (TEM) [10] (Fig.20.1a). Post cryopreservation, the lenticule collagen fibril architecture was found to be comparable to that of freshly extracted lenticules, with a well-preserved and aligned structure, without fragmented fibrils or areas of collagen disruption. This regular collagen structure and organization was also maintained after thawing (Fig. 20.1b). However, because of tissue hydration after cryopreservation, the lenticule collagen fibril density (CFD) was lower post cryopreservation (from 15.75 ± 1.56 to 12.05 ± 0.62, $p = 0.02$) although there was no significant change in the number of collagen fibrils ($p = 0.09$) [10]. Regular collagen architecture is one of the key factors in maintaining cornea transparency [13]. Therefore, the maintenance of regular cornea collagen architecture is important following cryopreservation, if the lenticule is to be considered for reimplantation.

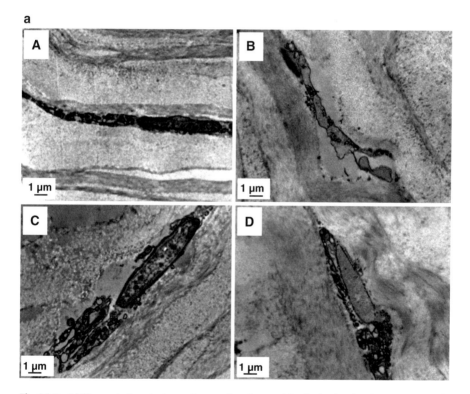

a

Fig. 20.1   (a) Transmission electron micrographs of stromal lenticule showing keratocytes. A, C: Fresh lenticule. B, D: Cryopreserved lenticule. A, B: Apoptotic keratocytes with chromatin condensation and fragmentation, apoptotic bodies, loss of cytoplasm, and cell shrinkage. C, D: Necrotic keratocyte, with incomplete nuclear membrane and vacuoles in the cytoplasm. Magnification, 8900×. (b) Transmission electron micrographs of the stromal lenticule showing collagen fibrils. A, C: Fresh lenticules. B, D: Cryopreserved lenticules. A, B: Transversal section of collagen fibrils. C, D: Longitudinal section of collagen fibrils. Magnification, 50,000× (Courtesy of Mohamed-Noriega et al. [10])

b

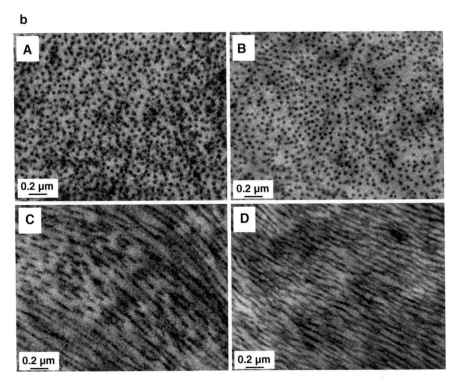

Fig. 20.1 (continued)

20.4 Apoptosis Detection

Following cryopreservation, there were significantly more TUNEL-positive cells and a proportional reduction in the number of DAPI-stained cells in the center of the lenticule compared to the periphery [10]. However, altogether, there were more TUNEL-positive cells located in the periphery than in the center of both fresh and cryopreserved lenticules [10]. This implied that the peripheral damage was produced by FS laser, although the keratocytes located in the center were more susceptible to damage during cryopreservation and thawing process.

20.5 In Vitro Cell Viability and Gene Expression Analysis

Viable keratocytes were able to be cultured from both fresh and cryopreserved lenticules, and there was no difference in cellular morphology or proliferation rates between both groups [10, 13, 14] (Fig. 20.2). This suggests that although dead keratocytes were seen using TEM and TUNEL assay, there were enough viable keratocytes within the cryopreserved lenticules that could be isolated and propagated.

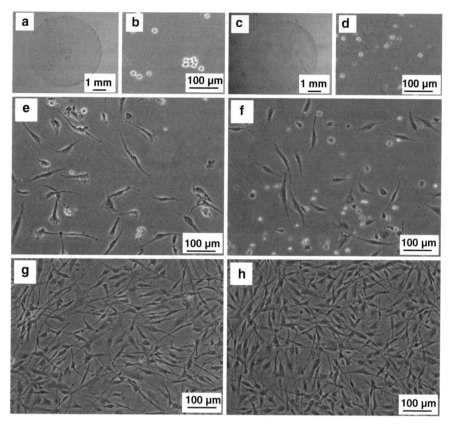

Fig. 20.2 Representative images of cultured keratocytes from ReLEx lenticules. (**a, b, e, g**) Fresh samples. (**c, d, f, h**) Cryopreserved samples. (**a, c**): ReLEx lenticules. (**b, d**) Free-floating stromal keratocytes following enzymatic digestion for at least 4 h in collagenase. (**e, f**) Attached kerato-cytes beginning to elongate into spindle-like fibroblastic cells by day 2 in culture. (**g, h**) Confluent stromal fibroblasts after 7 days in culture (Courtesy of et al. [10])

Gene expression demonstrated keratocyte-specific markers, human aldehyde dehy-drogenase 3A1 (ALDH3A1), and keratocan (KERA) to be found on both cells from fresh and cryopreserved keratocytes [10]. Both of these proteins are involved in the maintenance of corneal transparency [13, 14].

Hence, stromal lenticules extracted from ReLEx has been shown to remain via-ble after cryopreservation [10]. Although there was a decrease in CFD, the overall collagen architecture was preserved and there was good keratocyte viability. Keratocytes have been shown to be an important contributor for maintenance of corneal transparency, and this may be important if the lenticule is to be reimplanted in the future [13–17]. However, as corneal stromal buttons decellularized of kerato-cytes have been shown to be viable following host keratocyte migration [18], the maintenance of overall collagen structural integrity post cryopreservation may be the more important finding.

20.6   Lenticule Reimplantation

The concept of potential reversibility can have significant appeal to patients by offering them the reassurance of being able to restore their corneas to the preoperative state and also allowing other future treatment. Potential uses of lenticule reimplantation include the correction of iatrogenic corneal ectasia, where stromal volume is restored in areas of thinning. This may be combined with collagen cross-linking performed to both the lenticule and host cornea for further structural re-enforcement to further arrest the ectatic process [19]. It may also be used as a means of treating presbyopia, by reimplanting the autologous lenticule reshaped to a +1.5 or +2.0 D power, in the nondominant eye of a previously myopic patient who had undergone refractive surgery to near emmetropia, to create a state of monovision [20]. With informed consent and serology clearance, it may also be used as an allogenic biological intrastromal inlay in the same manner as a synthetic corneal refractive inlay that has demonstrated some promise in the treatment of presbyopia, yet obviating the issues of polymer biocompatibility and complications such as corneal melting, alteration in tear film thickness and corneal topography, corneal erosions, and peri-inlay deposits [21–24].

The proof of concept of the idea of autologous cryopreserved lenticule reimplantation has been demonstrated in rabbit and a long-term monkey model [25, 26]. In the rabbit model, it was demonstrated that lenticule reimplantation restored preoperative corneal thickness and caused minimal corneal haze and wound healing responses in the short term [25]. At 28 days post-reimplantation, the implanted corneas were indistinguishable from unoperated control eyes [25]. In the monkeys, the safety, efficacy, and long-term outcome of autologous, cryopreserved lenticule reimplantation following myopic correction were further evaluated, with an emphasis on determining the potential for reversibility with regard to restoration of corneal thickness, curvature, and refractive status [26].

The rabbits underwent −6.00D ReLEx (FLEx) correction in one eye with the contralateral eye used as unoperated controls [27]. Stromal lenticules were transferred on to rigid gas permeable (RGP) contact lenses (Bausch & Lomb) with careful attention to maintaining anatomical lenticular orientation. The contact lens was placed in a lens case and cryopreservation technique was similar as described above [10]. Reimplantation of the lenticule was carried out 28 days after initial ReLEx (FLEx) procedure.

Slit lamp photographs showed that corneal clarity progressively improved from day 3 to day 28 following lenticule reimplantation and on day 28 was comparable to before ReLEx (FLEx) surgery (Fig. 20.3a). This was matched by a commensurate reduction in interface reflectivity based on confocal microscopy measurements: The anterior and posterior border of the lenticule showed increased light reflectance and was acellular on day 3 after reimplantation. On day 14, the reflective layer at both interfaces was less prominent and keratocytes were visible, particularly at the posterior interface of the lenticule (Fig. 20.3b). The reflectivity level of the anterior and posterior borders were seen to decrease over the duration of the study, with the intensity of the anterior border decreasing from 117.09 ± 20.67 on day 3 to 83.73 ± 14.15 on day 28 and the posterior border decreasing from 105.15 ± 12.87 on

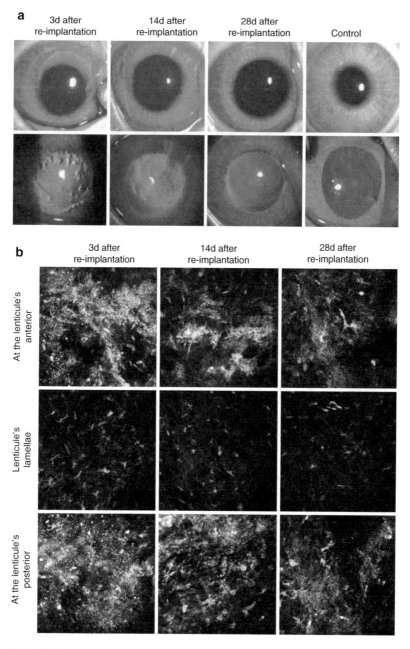

Fig. 20.3 (**a**) The top panel shows slit lamp photographs of the nonoperated cornea (control) and cornea on days 3, 14, and 28 after lenticule reimplantation. The bottom panel shows retro illumination photographs of the control and postoperative corneas. (**b**) In vivo confocal micrographs of the corneas on days 3, 14, and 28 after lenticule reimplantation. The top panel shows the anterior border of the lenticule within the reimplanted cornea. The middle panel shows the presence of quiescent keratocytes within the lenticule's lamellae. The bottom panel shows the posterior interface of the lenticule. Repopulation of the anterior and posterior borders of the lenticule occurs by day 28 (Courtesy of Angunawela et al. [25])

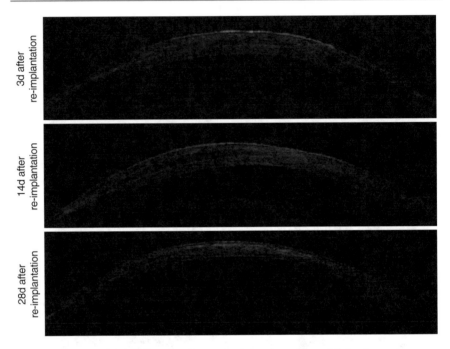

Fig. 20.4 Temporal AS-OCT images of postoperative corneas show resolving tissue edema over time (Courtesy of Angunawela et al. [25])

day 3 to 90.09 ± 14.10 on day 28. Significant difference ($p < 0.05$) was noted between day 3 and control and day 14 and control at both interfaces. The final keratometry following reimplantation was -0.6 ± 0.8 D from the preoperative correction. AS-OCT showed the corneas to be edematous compared to control eyes on day 3 after reimplantation but returned to normal at subsequent time points (Fig. 20.4).

Confocal microscopy also demonstrated resident keratocytes within the center of the lenticule, which remained quiescent and did not change in morphology and activity from day 3 to 28. There was repopulation of the anterior and posterior lenticular borders by day 28, with increased numbers of keratocytes appearing at the anterior and posterior border. There was no proliferating Ki67-positive cells noted and only a few apoptotic TUNEL-positive cells found within the lenticule on immunohistochemical staining. Together with positive staining for cellular actin as indicated by the relatively strong staining of phalloidin, which is a contractile cytoskeletal element found within the cell body, this implied that repopulation of the lenticular borders occurred through cell migration of adjacent keratocyte rather than from keratocyte proliferation. This is probably partly due to the fact that the lenticule itself contains a viable resident population of cells.

On immunohistochemical staining, no myofibroblasts or fibroblasts were detected in the reimplanted cornea, which was indicated by the absence of α-SMA. Both these cell types are implicated in scarring and haze formation in the cornea [27, 28]. Leukocyte integrin $\beta2$ (CD 18) was seen expressed by only a few cell and predominantly found at the interfaces of the lenticule; this is an inflammatory marker and mediator of polymorphonuclear leukocyte (PMN) migration within the corneal stroma. Tenascin-C, which is normally found in corneal epithelial cells and only found in corneal stroma after an injury, was detected within the lenticule and mainly along the anterior border. Fibronectin was expressed along the anterior and posterior borders of the lenticule on day 28. The weak healing stimulus, as seen by the minimal expression of fibronectin and tenascin-C, following lenticule reimplantation and the lack of inflammation are advantageous in maintaining corneal clarity and refractive accuracy following refractive stromal reimplantation procedures.

In the monkey model, 8 eyes were used to study long-term effect of ReLEx, 14 eyes for long-term effect of lenticule reimplantation, and 2 eyes as controls for immunohistochemical analysis [26]. The eyes underwent −6.00D ReLEx (FLEx) myopia correction and the storage and cryopreservation of the extracted lenticule were conducted as described before [10, 25]. Lenticule reimplantation was performed 4 months after ReLEx (FLEx) procedure. Corneal clarity was noted to progressively improve from 2.43 ± 0.53 at day 3 after reimplantation to 2.00 ± 0.58 at week 2, 1.07 ± 0.73 at week 4, and 0.21 ± 0.27 at week 8 and to stabilize at 0.14 ± 0.24 at week 16. There was no significant difference in the clarity of reimplanted corneas on weeks 8 and 16 compared to preoperated corneas. The effectiveness of this technique in reversing the refractive procedure was demonstrated by the restoration of corneal thickness, curvature, and refractive error indices to near preoperative values following lenticule reimplantation: AS-OCT showed significant difference in corneal thickness ($p < 0.001$) between the corneas pre- and post-ReLEx, but no significant difference between the corneas pre-ReLEx (425.05 ± 30.25 μm) and post-lenticule reimplantation (423.76 ± 36.67 μm). Cornea keratometry showed the cornea became flatter ($54.1 \pm 2.4D$) 16 weeks after ReLEx, but on week 16 post-reimplantation of lenticule, corneas were steepened centrally and keratometry values were similar to preoperative corneas ($58.0 \pm 1.2D$ vs $58.6 \pm 2.1D$, $p = 0.506$). There was no significant difference in the corneal spherical error pre-ReLEx and post-reimplantation; the spherical error before ReLEx was $-1.64 \pm 0.56D$, becoming $+4.29 \pm 0.86D$ at week 16 after −6.00D myopic correction ($p < 0.001$) which indicates that the eyes were $-0.07 \pm 0.45D$ from the intended correction. The refraction was restored to $-1.64 \pm 0.35D$ at week 16 after lenticule reimplantation ($p = 0.891$).

Confocal microscopy showed that keratocytes were visible at both interfaces of the reimplanted lenticule on weeks 8 and 16. Activated and elongated keratocytes within the center of the lenticule were observed on week 8, but by week 16, most of the keratocytes appeared normal and quiescent and resembled those found in the preoperative corneal stroma. There was only a mild corneal wound healing reaction with both fibronectin and tenascin predominantly present along the anterior and posterior interfaces of the reimplanted lenticule on week 8 and their expression diminishing by week 16 (Fig. 20.5). Collagen type I, the predominant collagen type in cornea stroma, was uniformly expressed in full thickness of both the control and postoperative corneas, indicating normal collagen expression, maintaining corneal

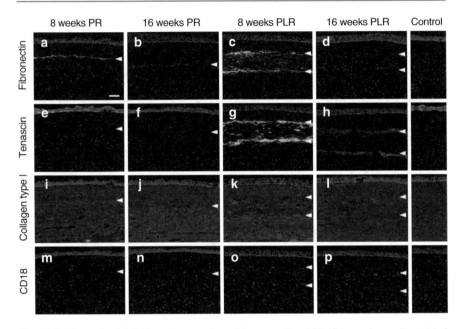

Fig. 20.5 Expression of fibronectin, tenascin, collagen type I and CD18 in post-operative central corneas. (**a–d**) Fibronectin predominantly appeared along the laser incision site or lenticular inter-face. The expression was reduced over time after either ReLEx or refractive lenticule re-implantation. (**e–h**) Tenascin was absent along the flap interface on week 8 and 16 following ReLEx, but was present along the borders of the stromal lenticule after re-implantation. The inten-sity of the staining was attenuated over time. (**i–l**) Collagen type I was expressed uniformly in the full thickness of comeal stroma. No significant anomaly in collagen arrangement was observed in the corneas post-ReLEx and post-reimplantation. (M-P) CD18-positive cells were not seen in all post-operative corneas. Unoperated corneas were used as control. *Arrowheads* indicate the loca-tion of the laser incision site or lenticular interface. *PR* post-ReLEx, *PLR* post-lenticule re-implantation. Scale 50 μm (Courtesy of Riau et al. [26])

transparency (Fig. 20.5). Leukocyte integrin β2 (CD 18) was not expressed in post-ReLEx and post-reimplantation corneas (Fig. 20.5). No proliferating Ki67-positive cells and no apoptotic TUNEL-positive cells were found within the lenticule. There was relatively strong staining of phalloidin in the anterior and posterior portions of the lenticule on week 8 post-reimplantation (Fig. 20.6). There was no myofibro-blasts detected in the central cornea (indicated by the absence of α-SMA) at weeks 8 and 16 after ReLEx and lenticule reimplantation (Fig. 20.7).

Current clinical methods for stromal volume restoration are mainly limited to various techniques of anterior lamellar keratoplasty which involves surgical dissec-tion and replacement of the host stroma with donor stromal tissue [29]. These are technically and surgically demanding and also carry risk of graft rejection [30]. Epikeratophakia was another method of stromal volume restoration technique in vogue in the 1990s, which involved the removal of host corneal epithelium and fixa-tion by suture of a cryolathed donor corneal lenticule on to the Bowman's mem-brane, as an overlay allograft over which the host epithelium would heal [31, 32].

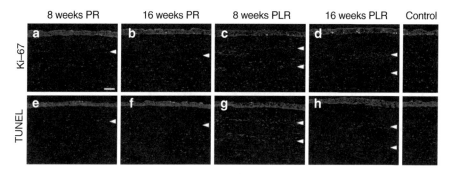

Fig. 20.6 Immunofluorescent staining of Ki-67, TUNEL and phalloidin in post-operative central corneas. (**a–d**) Ki-67 positive cells (*green*) were not found in the comeal stroma on week 8 and 16 after ReLEx and refractive lenticule re-implantation. (**e–h**) Similarly, presence of TUNEL-positive cells (*green*) was not detected in the corneal stroma. In pane **a–h**, F-actin marker (*red*), phalloidin, was observed in the laser incision site or lenticular interface. Its presence was attenuated over time. Nuclei were counterstained using DAPI (*blue*). Unoperated corneas were used as control. *Arrowheads* indicate the location of the laser incision site or lenticular interface. *PR* post-ReLEx, *PLR* post-lenticule re-implantation. Scale bar. 50 µm (Courtesy of Riau et al. [26])

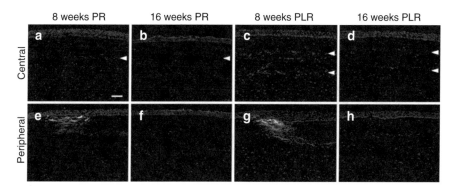

Fig 20.7 Expression of α-smooth muscle actin (α-SMA) in the post-operative central corneas and peripheral flaps. (**a–d**) α-SMA (*green*), a marker of myofibroblasts, was not present in the central corneas on week 8 and 16 after both ReLEx and refractive lenticule re-implantation. (**e–h**) α-SMA (*green*) was expressed at the flap periphery and co-localized with F-actin (*red*) subepithelially on week 8 post-ReLEx and lenticule re-implantation, but was absent 16 weeks after both surgical procedures. In pane **a–h**, α-SMA (*green*) was double immunostained with F-actin marker (*red*), phalloidin. Nuclei were counterstained using DAPI (*blue*). *Arrowheads* indicate the location of the laser incision site or lenticular interface. *PR* post-ReLEx, *PLR* post-lenticule re-implantation. Scale bar: 50 µm (Courtesy of Riau et al. [26])

However, the failure to widely adopt this technique resulted from imprecise refractive outcomes and postoperative complications such as interface scarring. In contrast, ReLEx with lenticule reimplantation has significant advantage in terms of lamellar accuracy and refractive correction, as well as when used in autologous implant, circumventing the risk of tissue rejection and need for prolonged topical immunosuppression postoperatively. The relative absence of inflammation and wound healing processes [25, 26] as a result of it being an intrastromal procedure results in less interface haze, compared to epikeratophakia, which involves a surface-related wound healing procedure.

20.7   Potential for Treatment of Presbyopia

The feasibility of performing a secondary refractive surgical procedure, i.e., LASIK, in order to achieve a monovision correction in patients with presbyopia, who have previously undergone ReLEx for myopic correction, has been demonstrated in a rabbit model of SMILE [33]. Corneal haze and inflammatory cells were seen at the anterior and posterior borders of the reimplanted lenticule on in vivo confocal microscopy early after surgery, which gradually resolved over the 5-week follow-up period. This observation was confirmed by slit-lamp examination, where progressive improvement in corneal clarity was observed. No complications such as diffuse lamellar keratitis were noted in all cases. Immunohistochemistry staining of fibronectin, CD11b, Ki67, and TUNEL showed no difference from control corneas 5 weeks after lenticule reimplantation.

Anterior segment OCT showed transient thickening of the corneas following lenticule reimplantation and post-LASIK, likely attributable to inflammatory response and corneal edema. The reimplanted lenticule appeared thinner after excimer laser ablation of the anterior stroma. The anterior and posterior stromal-lenticular interfaces were visualized on confocal microscopy, and increased reflectance and acellularity in both planes were observed 1 week after implantation. Keratocyte repopulation was seen as early as 3 weeks post-reimplantation. Following LASIK, a highly reflective and acellular layer with interspersed particles was seen at the anterior interface, consistent with the excimer laser-ablated stromal plane. There was no significant difference in the reflectivity level of the interface between eyes that underwent LASIK post-SMILE vs. those that underwent LASIK alone ($p=0.310$), and there was also similar patterns and expression levels of fibronectin, as well as similar number of inflammatory cells ($p=0.304$) and apoptotic cells ($p=0.198$). These results suggest that there are no significant differences in the corneal tissue response and development of early postoperative corneal haze after performing LASIK on corneas that have previously undergone SMILE and subsequent lenticule reimplantation, in comparison with virgin eyes.

20.8   Potential Use of Lenticule in Human

With increasing number of eyes undergoing ReLEx SMILE and the extracted lenticule as a by-product, tissue banks have been set up to preserve these lenticules on a long-term basis using cryopreservation. In the first report on a human, an allogeneic lenticule obtained by SMILE from a myopic donor was implanted into a young individual for correction of high hypermetropia secondary to aphakia [34]. A pocket lamellar incision was created with the VisuMax®, the upper interface was then separated and donor lenticule inserted through the small incision. Retinoscopy refraction at 1 year was +7.50 −3.00×150, a spherical equivalent reduction of 5.52D, and mean keratometric power increased by 2.91D. Only 50 % of the intended correction was achieved due to posterior surface changes (posterior surface elevation changed significantly with a central bulge into the anterior chamber) and epithelial remodeling. However, no adverse side effects were observed over the 1-year postoperative period validating the previous monkey and rabbit studies.

Subsequently, a second study on lower hyperopia using cryopreserved lenticules has shown promising results in terms of safety, efficacy, and reproducibility [35]. In a clinical series on hyperopic patients, a technique of lenticular implantation was used (FS laser intrastromal lenticular implantation (FILI)) whereby a VisuMax® FS laser was used to create a 7.5-mm-diameter pocket at a depth of 160-µm and 4-mm superior incision. The lenticules were cryopreserved as previously described above with the exception of replacement of bovine serum albumin with human tissue culture media, to reduce the risk of zoonotic transmission [10]. The mean period of cryopreservation of the lenticules was 96 days (19–178 days). As previously hypothesized by Barraquer [36], the cornea was made steeper by the addition of a lenticule of known thickness and power into a pocket created in a patient's cornea. The incision was opened with a Seibel spatula and the plane of the pocket dissected. The cryopreserved lenticule was then marked in the center and inserted into the pocket, aligning the center with the papillary center. A depth of 160 µm was chosen for implantation in all patients due to uncertainty in refractive outcomes and the novelty of the nomograms and also to ensure the surgeon could have adequate tissue in the cap for later enhancement with surface ablation if required (Fig. 20.8).

All eyes had central corneal steepening with a mean change in anterior keratometry of 3.5D in the central 3-mm zone. There was an average 0.33D flattening of posterior corneal curvature in all eyes, which was seen more in thicker lenticules compared with thinner ones (Fig. 20.9). The postoperative Q values in all the eyes became more negative (mean Q value changed from −0.38 to −0.89), suggesting a hyperprolate shift. This change in asphericity after FILI is expected after tissue addition, although the observed change was not seen as much after hyperopic LASIK [37]. The shape of the cornea after tissue additive procedure is more natural compared with tissue subtractive procedures like photorefractive keratectomy and LASIK, which steepen the cornea by ablating the mid-peripheral tissue. The correction of hyperopia by laser procedures can be associated with significant regression in higher degrees of refractive errors and induction of higher-order aberrations (HOAs) [38, 39]. The total HOAs after FILI remained within normal acceptable values and did not show a significant increase postoperatively ($p > 0.05$). The procedure was predictable in the treatment of moderate hyperopia with all eyes having residual spherical equivalence within ±1.0D, although the results were not highly accurate for treatment of very high hyperopia, e.g., aphakia: the aphakic eye had residual spherical equivalence +4.1D.

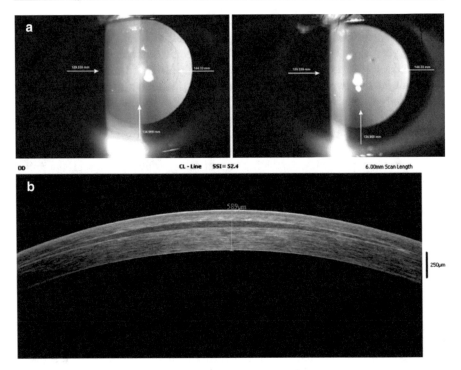

Fig. 20.8 (**a**) Serial digital photographs (16×) of a 32-year-old woman operated for +6.5D hyperopia in the right eye with FILI. Photographs were taken on day 15 and 6 months after the operation. Distance from edge of the lenticule to limbus was measured at 3 points and verified at every visit to check for centering and any shift in position. (**b**) Six-month postoperative anterior segment optical coherence tomography of an eye treated for +6.5D hyperopia showing a clear and well-centered lenticule (Courtesy of Ganesh et al. [35])

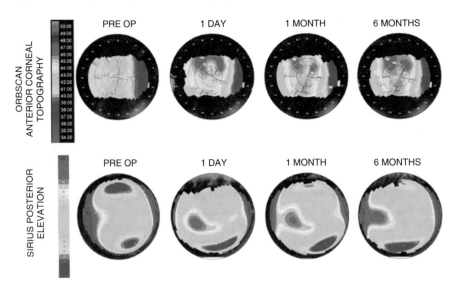

Fig. 20.9 Orbscan anterior corneal surface topography (*top*) and Sirius posterior elevation (*bottom*) over the 6-month postoperative course after FILI for eye with +6.5 D hyperopia (Courtesy of Ganesh et al. [35])

Conclusion

The cryopreservation technique described seems to be a safe method of long-term storage of refractive lenticules extracted after ReLEx for use in human subjects. The preliminary results show that reimplantation of the lenticules is a feasible technique for restoring stromal volume after myopic ReLEx and for treating low levels of hyperopia. Further studies examining lenticule reshaping into a small optic presbyopic lenticules are currently underway. For allograft lenticules, informed consent and full serological evaluation of donors similar to that required in eye bank cornea tissue donors for corneal transplantation would be required.

References

1. Blum M, Kunert K, Schroder M, Sekundo W (2010) Femtosecond lenticule extraction for the correction of myopia: preliminary 6-month results. Graefes Arch Clin Exp Ophthalmol 248:1019–1027
2. Sekundo W, Kunert K, Russmann C et al (2008) First efficacy and safety study of femtosecond lenticule extraction for the correction of myopia: six month results. J Cataract Refract Surg 34:1513–1520
3. Sekundo W, Kunert KS, Blum M (2011) Small incision corneal refractive surgery using the small incision lenticule extraction (SMILE) procedure for the correction of myopia and myopic astigmatism: results of a 6 month prospective study. Br J Ophthalmol 95:335–339
4. Shah R, Shah S, Sengupta S (2011) Results of small incision lenticule extraction: all-in-one femtosecond laser refractive surgery. J Cataract Refract Surg 37:127–137
5. Capella JA, Kaufmann HE, Robbins JE (1965) Preservation of viable corneal tissue. Cryobiology 2:116–121
6. Eastcott HH, Cross AG, Leigh AG, North DP (1954) Preservation of corneal grafts by freezing. Lancet 266:237–239
7. Oh JY, Kim MK, Lee HJ, Ko JH, We WR, Le JH (2009) Comparative observation of freeze-thaw-induced damage in pig, rabbi, and human corneal stroma. Vet Ophthalmol 12:50–56
8. Halberstadt M, Böhnke M, Athmann S, Hagenah M (2003) Cryopreservation of human donor corneas with dextran. Invest Ophthalmol Vis Sci 44:5110–5115
9. Oh JY, Lee HJ, Khwarg SI, Wee WR (2010) Corneal cell viability and structure after transcorneal freezing-thawing in the human cornea. Clin Ophthalmol 4:477–480
10. Mohamed-Noriega K, Toh KP, Poh R et al (2011) Cornea lenticule viability and structural integrity after refractive lenticule extraction (ReLEx) and cryopreservation. Mol Vis 17:3437–3449
11. Hunt CJ (2011) Cryopreservation of human stem cells for clinical application: a review. Transfus Med Hemother 38:107–123
12. Hayakawa J, Joyal EG, Gildner JF et al (2010) 5 % dimethyl sulfoxide (DMSO) and pentastarch improves cryopreservation of cord blood cells over 10 % DMSO. Transfusion 50:2158–2166
13. Hassell JR, Birk D (2010) The molecular basis of corneal transparency. Exp Eye Res 91:326–335
14. Pei Y, Reins RY, McDermott AM (2006) Aldehyde dehydrogenase (ALSH) 3A1 expression by the human keratocyte and its repair phenotypes. Exp Eye Res 83:1063–1073
15. West-Mays JA, Dqivedi DJ (2006) The keratocyte: corneal stromal cell with variable repair phenotypes. Int J Biochem Cell Biol 38:1625–1631
16. Jester JV (2008) Corneal crystalline and development of cellular transparency. Semin Cell Dev Biol 19:82–93
17. Fini ME, Stramer BM (2005) How the cornea heals: cornea-specific repair mechanisms affecting surgical outcomes. Cornea 24:S2–S11

18. Amanos S, Shimomura N, Yokoo S, Araki-Sasaki K, Yamagami S (2008) Decellularizing corneal stroma using N2 gas. Mol Vis 14:878–882
19. Caster AI, Friess DW, Schwendeman FJ (2010) Incidence of epithelial ingrowth in primary and retreatment laser in situ keratomileusis. J Cataract Refract Surg 36:97–101
20. Goldberg DB (2001) Laser in situ keratomileusis monovision. J Cataract Refract Surg 27:1449–1455
21. Waring GO 4th, Klyce SD (2011) Corneal inlays for the treatment of presbyopia. Int Ophthalmol Clin 51:51–62
22. Dexl AK, Ruckhofer J, Riha W, Hohensinn M, Rueckl T et al (2011) Central and peripheral corneal iron deposits after implantation of a small-aperture corneal inlay for correction of presbyopia. J Refract Surg 27:876–880
23. Evans MD, Prakasam RK, Vaddavalli PK, Hughes TC, Knower W et al (2011) A perfluoropolyether corneal inlay for the correction of refractive error. Biomaterials 32:3158–3165
24. Mulet ME, Alio JL, Knorz MC (2009) Hydrogel intracorneal inlays for the correction of hyperopia: outcomes and complications after 5 years of follow-up. Ophthalmology 116:1455–1460
25. Angunawela RI, Riau A, Chaurasia SS et al (2012) Refractive lenticule re-implantation after myopic ReLEx: a feasibility study of stromal restoration after refractive surgery in a rabbit model. Invest Ophthalmol Vis Sci 53(8):4975–4985
26. Riau AK, Angunawela RI, Chaurasia SS, Lee WS, Tan DT, Mehta JS (2013) Reversible femtosecond laser assisted myopia correction: a non-human primate study of lenticule re-implantation after refractive lenticule extraction. PLoS ONE 8(6), e67058. doi:10.1371/journal.pone.0067058
27. Wilson SE (2002) Analysis of the keratocyte apoptosis, keratocyte proliferation, and myofibroblast transformation responses after photorefractive keratectomy and laser in situ keratomileusis. Trans Am Ophthalmol Soc 100:411–433
28. Netto MV, Mohan RR, Sinha S, Sharma A, Dupps W, Wilson SE (2006) Stromal haze, myofibroblasts, and surface irregularity after PRK. Exp Eye Res 82:788–797
29. Bromley JG, Randleman JB (2010) Treatment strategies for cornea ectasia. Curr Opin Ophthalmol 21:255–258
30. Klebe S, Coster DJ, Williams KA (2009) Rejection and acceptance of corneal allografts. Curr Opin Organ Transplant 14:4–9
31. Kaminski SL, Biowski R, Koyuncu D, Lukas JR, Grabner G (2003) Ten year follow-up of epikeratophakia for the correction of high myopia. Ophthalmology 110:2147–2152
32. Spitznas M, Eckert J, Frising M, Eter N (2002) Long-term functional and topographic results seven years after epikeratophakia for keratoconus. Graefes Arch Clin Exp Ophthalmol 240:639–643
33. Lim CHL, Riau AK, Lwin NC, Chaurasia SS, Tan DT, Mehta JS (2013) LASIK following small incision lenticule extraction (SMILE) lenticule re-implantation: a feasibility study of a novel method for treatment of presbyopia. PLoS ONE 8(12), e83046
34. Pradhan KR, Reisntein DZ, Carp GI et al (2013) Femtosecond laser-assisted keyhole endokeratophakia: correction of hyperopia by implantation of an allogeneic lenticule obtained by SMILE from a myopic donor. J Refract Surg 29:777–782
35. Ganesh S, Brar S, Rao PA (2014) Cryopreservation of extracted corneal lenticules after small incision lenticule extraction for potential use in human subjects. Cornea 33(12):1355–1362
36. Barraquer JI (1993) Refractive corneal surgery. Experience and considerations. An Inst Barraquer 24:113–118
37. Chen CC, Izadshenas A, Rana MA et al (2002) Corneal asphericity after hyperopic laser in situ keratomileusis. J Cataract Refract Surg 28:1539–1545
38. Goker S, Kahvecioglu C (1998) Laser in situ keratomileusis to correct hyperopia from +4.25 to +8.00 diopters. J Refract Surg 14:26–30
39. Pesudovs K (2005) Wavefront aberration outcomes of LASIK for high myopia and hyperopia. J Refract Surg 21:S508–S512

SMILE in Special Cases

21

Moones Abdalla and Osama Ibrahim

Contents

As mentioned earlier in this book, SMILE has shown great efficacy and accuracy in normal corneas, having its unique and special advantages over any other refractive techniques, being flapless and less invasive. Furthermore, the ability to tailor and center the procedure as required within the cornea, together with better biomechanical stability [1], made SMILE a reasonable technique to deal with special cases which will be discussed in this chapter.

Electronic supplementary material The online version of this chapter (doi:10.1007/978-3-319-18530-9_21) contains supplementary material, which is available to authorized users.

M. Abdalla (✉) • O. Ibrahim
Roayah Vision Correction Center, Alexandria, Egypt

Alexandria University, Alexandria, Egypt

International FemtoLASIK Centre (IFLC), Cairo, Egypt
e-mail: moones.abdalla@gmail.com

© Springer International Publishing Switzerland 2015
W. Sekundo (ed.), *Small Incision Lenticule Extraction (SMILE):*
Principles, Techniques, Complication Management, and Future Concepts,
DOI 10.1007/978-3-319-18530-9_21

21.1   Combined SMILE and Cross-Linking (CXL)

Moones Abdalla, Ahmad El Massry, Assem Zahran,
Eman El Maghraby, and Osama Ibrahim

Theoretically, SMILE has biomechanical advantages over LASIK because it does not involve the creation of a flap and leaves the stroma over the lenticule almost untouched, making it a procedure with minimal alterations of corneal biomechanics [2, 3]. However, there are not many published studies regarding these biomechanical benefits of SMILE.

In SMILE, the refractive stromal tissue removal takes place in deeper stroma, leaving the stronger anterior stroma intact, thus leaving the cornea with greater tensile strength than LASIK for any given refractive correction [4, 5]. Based on Randleman's data, the model predicted that the postoperative tensile strength after SMILE was approximately 10 % higher than PRK and 25 % higher than LASIK [6].

We anticipated that combining SMILE with intrastromal collagen cross-linking (CXL) would add to the safety, predictability, and stability of SMILE alone when conventional laser vision correction is not favored because of suspicious topography and or thin corneas . Furthermore, we reasoned that combining CXL with SMILE in eyes with forme fruste keratoconus (FFKC) or early keratoconus could strengthen the cornea to stop the progression of the ectatic disease while meeting patient demands for improving unaided vision. This prospective study included 34 eyes of 18 patients suffering from myopic astigmatism, with topography not suitable for LASIK or diagnosis of FFKC, moreover we included patients with a stable refraction and topographic findings for at least 1 year, CDVA>0.7 (Snellen decimal), central corneal thickness >460 μm, and patient age >21 years.

21.1.1 Surgical Technique

SMILE was performed using VisuMax® 500 kHz laser (Carl Zeiss Meditec AG, Germany). All cases had a 100 μm cap and a minimum of 300 μm of residual stromal bed. Intra-pocket injection of isotonic riboflavin three times with a 5 min interval was followed by 5 min of UV irradiation using 18 mW/cm². Biomechanical stability was assessed using the Corvis® ST (Oculus GmbH, Germany), measuring and correlating IOP and deformation amplitude.

21.1.2 Results

Mean patient age was $29.4 \pm 5.63(22–35)$. Mean preoperative refraction was -3.97 ± 1.87 D sphere (range -6.0 to -1.25) and -2.85 D cylinder (range -0.75 to -4.25). Mean postoperative spherical refraction was -0.14 ± 0.73 D (range -1.25 to

Fig. 21.1 Uncorrected visual acuity change (decimal) during the follow-up time

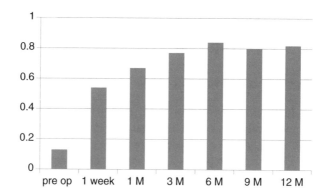

+1.5) and mean astigmatism was −0.38±0.45 D. Seventy-two percent was within ±0.5 and 89 % within ±1.0 D at the end of the follow-up. The change in the mean UCVA is shown in Fig. 21.1. Delayed recovery of visual outcome was noticed due to haze, which was found to improve 1–3 months after surgery.

21.1.3 Topographic Changes

Example 1 (Fig. 21.2) Example 2 (Fig. 21.3)   A 24-year-old male patient having −5 sphere and −1 cylinder with a family history of keratoconus a family history of keratoconus; a factor which was considered to be a contraindication for LASIK. As a result, the decision of performing SMILE and CXL was taken.

Postoperatively, a further flattening was noticed, which we felt was due to the progressive effect of CXL and presumambly resulting in more stability over time. This pattern of progressive flatening was obseved in about 35 % of cases.

Using Corvis® technology, mean deformation amplitude was 1.38 mm ±0.29 pre-op. One month after surgery, the mean deformation amplitude decreased to 1.19 mm ±0.29. No significant change over follow-up period occurred thereafter (for details, see Videos 2 and 3).

All cases treated so far showed topographic stability over the follow-up period up to 1 year. Figure 21.4 shows a Scheimpflug image of the cornea after combined SMILE and CXL.

In conclusion, simultaneous SMILE and in-the-pocket cross-linking might be a safe predictable and stable treatment option in patients where conventional laser refractive surgery is contraindicated. A delayed visual recovery associated with a transient haze formation was a temporary drawback of this procedure with the CXL regimen as described above. Further follow-up, larger samples, and different ribo-flavin preparations as well as application techniques have to be studied to ensure the best possible outcome of this combined procedure. Moreover, at present, we don't know the boundaries of this approach: this needs to be elucidated in further prospective studies as shown in the following case report below.

21.2 Combined SMILE and CXL for Post-Intracorneal Ring Implantation (ICR) for Progressive Keratoconus: A Case Report

Moones Abdalla, Eman El Maghrabi, and Osama Ibrahim

In keratoconus patients who underwent previous CXL, performing SMILE would remove cross-linked tissue, so intra-pocket CXL was performed again for fear of progression and recurrence of keratoconus.

This is a case report of a 29-year-old female suffering from bilateral KC and had ICRs implanted in both eyes 11 months ago. The UCVA in her left eye was 0.3 with a manifest refraction of −1.5 to 5.0 at 65. This refraction was stable for 7 months and the CDVA was = 0.8. Despite the temporary stabilization of the disease by ICRs, the patient was unhappy with his unaided vision. A rigid contact lens was not an option. Patient's topography is shown in Fig. 21.5.

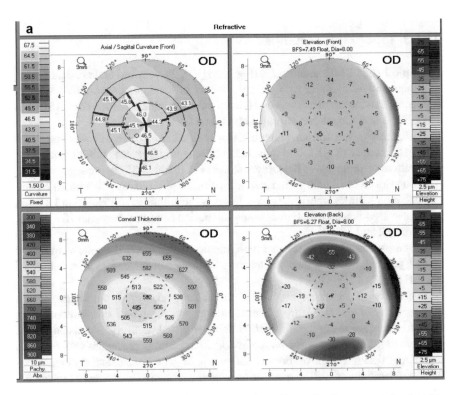

Fig. 21.2 (a) Pentacam® image of a 22-year-old male seeking refractive surgery showing thin cornea with inferotemporal steepening that was considered a contraindication to LASIK. Thus, a combined SMILE and CXL was performed. (b) Pentacam® of the same patient 3 months postoperatively showing topographic stability and no evidence of ectasia, which was noticed in all our cases

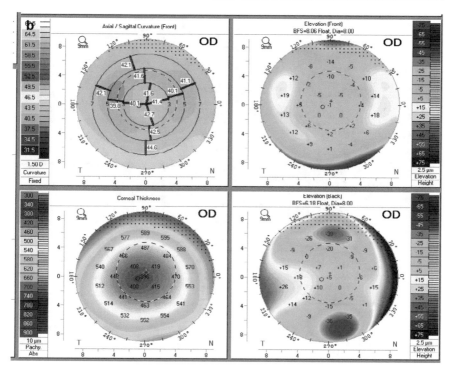

Fig. 21.2 (continued)

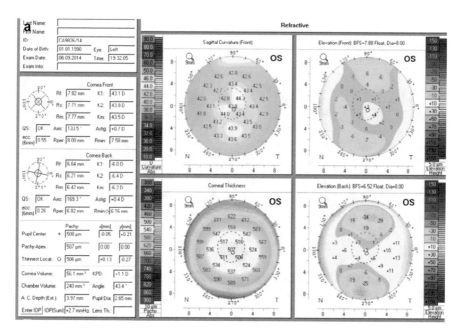

Fig. 21.3 (**a**) This depicts the irregular topography of the patient's left eye. Notably, the pachymetry map and the posterior float appear regular. (**b**) One month postoperative topography: inferior steepening was noticed. (**c**) Three months after surgery, the anterior cornea is flatter and thinner

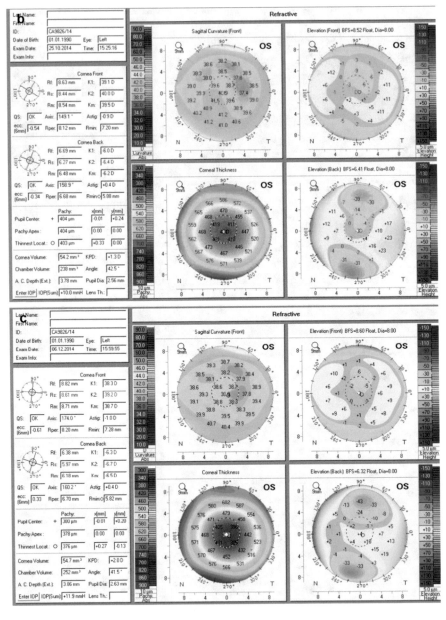

Fig. 21.3 (continued)

Correcting residual refractive error after ICR can be challenging. Topography-guided PRK is an option but is not suitable for correction of higher errors [19, 20]. SMILE is an option to correct residual high errors post-ICR cases, but it needs meticulous presurgical planning to place the lenticule within the ring segments.

Fig. 21.4 Notice the CXL demarcation line in the cornea after combined SMILE and CXL

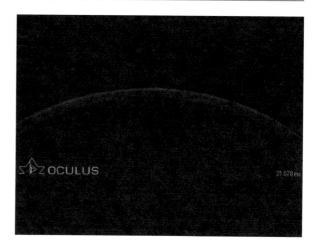

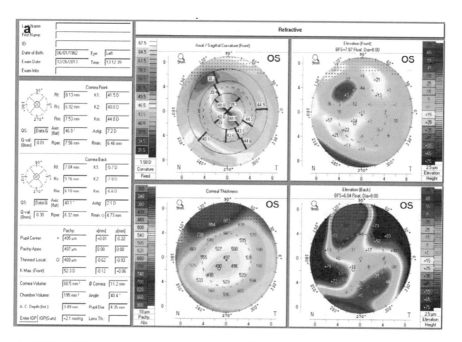

Fig. 21.5 (**a**) Scheimpflug image showing topographic results post-ICR, but before SMILE. (**b**) Laser settings for SMILE in keratoconus with ICRs

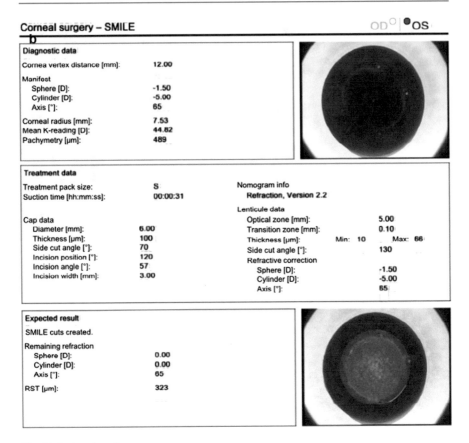

Corneal surgery – SMILE   OD ○ | ● OS

b

Diagnostic data			
Cornea vertex distance [mm]:	12.00		
Manifest			
Sphere [D]:	-1.50		
Cylinder [D]:	-5.00		
Axis [°]:	65		
Corneal radius [mm]:	7.53		
Mean K-reading [D]:	44.82		
Pachymetry [µm]:	489		

Treatment data					
Treatment pack size:	S		Nomogram info		
Suction time [hh:mm:ss]:	00:00:31		Refraction, Version 2.2		
			Lenticule data		
Cap data			Optical zone [mm]:		5.00
Diameter [mm]:	6.00		Transition zone [mm]:		0.10
Thickness [µm]:	100		Thickness [µm]:	Min: 10	Max: 66
Side cut angle [°]:	70		Side cut angle [°]:		130
Incision position [°]:	120		Refractive correction		
Incision angle [°]:	57		Sphere [D]:		-1.50
Incision width [mm]:	3.00		Cylinder [D]:		-5.00
			Axis [°]:		65

Expected result			
SMILE cuts created.			
Remaining refraction			
Sphere [D]:	0.00		
Cylinder [D]:	0.00		
Axis [°]:	65		
RST [µm]:	323		

Fig. 21.5 (continued)

21.2.1 Treatment Parameters

Treatment parameters were adjusted to the area between the ICRs. Therefore, unlike in the standard SMILE surgery, the optical zone was chosen to be 5 mm, and the cap had a total diameter of 6 mm. Further parameters are shown in the Fig. 21.5b. The energy settings were set quite low at level 25 (appr. 125nJ) and the spot/track distance reduced to 3 µm for the lamellar cuts and 2 µm for the vertical cuts. The centration was aimed exactly in-between the ICRs.

21.2.2 Surgical Procedure

The surgery is briefly summarized in Fig. 21.6a–c (for details, also see enclosed video). Noticeably, the centration was quite easy, because the initial tunnels for the ICRs implantation were performed with the same VisuMax® laser.

Fig. 21.6 (**a**) The applanation and the lenticule are perfectly centered between the ICRs. The ICRs are easily identified because of the positioning holes. (**b**) The cap overlies the ICRs, but being 100 μm thick is superficial enough not to interfere with the old ICR tunnel. A 3 mm opening incision is fashioned in the superonasal quadrant. (**c**) A snapshot of the lenticule extraction

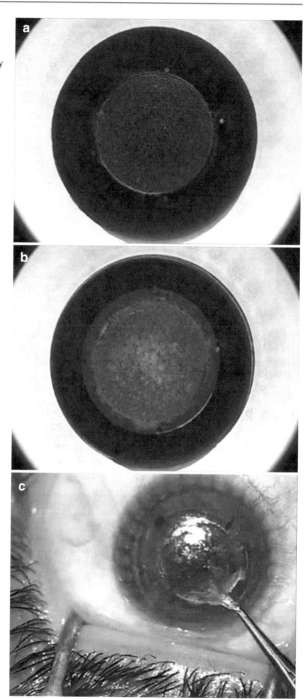

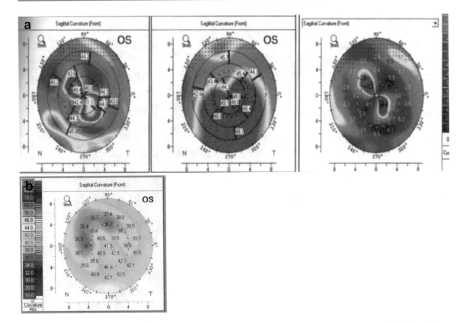

Fig. 21.7 (**a**) Immediate post-op differential topography (sagittal map) shows an effective reduction of astigmatism (from left to right: pre-op, post-op, and differential topography). (**b**) Three months after SMILE, there is a further regularization of the anterior surface resulting in the UCVA = 0.8

21.2.3 Results

Three months after SMILE, the patient has reached the preoperative BCVA (= 0.8) unaided.

21.3 SMILE for Post-Penetrating Keratoplasty Myopia and Astigmatism

Tamer Masoud, Moones Abdalla, Ibrahim Ahmed, and Osama Ibrahim

Despite the high incidence of obtaining clear corneal grafts and improved surgical techniques, postoperative corneal toricity and high myopia after penetrating keratoplasty (PKP) are a major limitation of visual outcome. The incidence of high astigmatism following keratoplasty varies from 10 to 30 % and is higher after PKP for keratoconus [7]. The unpredictable nature of corneal wound healing and the biomechanical response to surgery can lead to postoperative refractive surprises [8].

In LASIK for post-PKP errors, flap creation may induce astigmatism and higher-order aberrations [9, 10] because the flap itself is subject to shape changes induced by the vertical circumferential keratotomy of flap creation. This effect is magnified when the cut is through graft/host scar tissue. Furthermore, the risk of developing post-LASIK ectasia increases in patients with PKP for keratoconus, thick flaps, and deep laser ablation [11].

In SMILE, only a small vertical incision is made without the creation of a flap, minimizing trauma to the corneal surface if compared with other surgical procedures (PRK or LASIK) [12–15] which helps to preserve the graft's healing scar, avoiding the more peripheral, possibly diseased cornea.

SMILE in post-PKP cases has the advantage of centration of the lenticule within the graft, avoiding cutting in the previous incision scar tissue giving better prediction of treatment results. Furthermore, patients with preexisting keratoconus could have a higher risk of recurrence of keratoconus if the flap cut is in the recipient cornea.

Our study was conducted with the following inclusion criteria:

- Clear central cornea
- Corrected distance visual acuity (CDVA) of ≥ 0.5
- Minimal corneal thickness not less than 500 μm
- Maximum keratometric readings <55 D
- Spherical equivalent >−5 D
- Stable graft for more than 1 year without any signs of rejection
- All sutures should be removed at least 3 months before the procedure
- Duration after PKP ≥ 18 months
- Graft diameter more than 6 mm

Thirteen eyes of 13 patients with previous PKP, and residual myopic astigmatism were enrolled in the study. Pentacam imaging and thickness measurements were within the acceptable range for laser vision correction. The procedure and its possible advantages and hazards were explained to the patients, and an informed consent was obtained from each of them. Preoperatively, manifest refraction (MR), uncorrected distance visual acuity (UDVA), and corrected distance visual acuity (CDVA) were recorded. Intraoperatively, the cap and the lenticule diameters were calculated so that they are centered within the graft. The other parameters (optical zone, transition zone, and minimal thickness of the lenticule) were based on the degree of the refractive error, thinnest location of the graft, and the residual stromal depth under the cap. The same preoperative measurements (MR, UDVA, and CDVA) were obtained and recorded postoperatively at 1 month, 3 months, and 6 months. Standard graphs for reporting refractive procedures were used [16–18].

21.3.1 Example of Treatment Parameters

The treatment zone is chosen to be 5.4 mm and the cap 6.0 mm. All other parameters are identical to the abovementioned settings for pos- ICR SMILE.

21.3.2 Surgical Procedure

The surgery is briefly summarized in Fig. 21.8a, b (for details, also see enclosed video).

Fig. 21.8 (**a**) The post-PKP cornea is carefully applanated. The host-graft junction can be easily appreciated at this snapshot image. (**b**) The lenticule, the cap, and the opening incision are confined to the graft

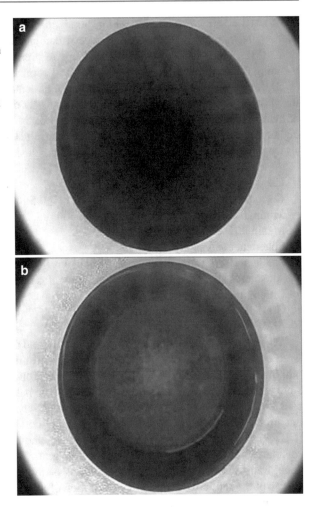

21.3.3 Results

Mean preoperative refraction was -4.54 ± 1.46 D sphere (range -8.75 to -1.25) and -4.65 D cylinder (range -1.5 to -7.0). Mean postoperative sphere was -0.56 ± 0.73 D (range -1.75 to $+1.5$) and mean astigmatism was -0.98 ± 0.45 D (up to -3.5). Figure 21.9a–c displays the visual results.

It was noticed that postoperative topographic cylinder was almost double the number of manifest refraction in most cases. Figure 21.10 shows a differential map of an uncomplicated case.

One eye encountered buttonhole in the cap intraoperatively due to irregular topography. We observed that a cornea with an irregular bow tie pattern with steep and flat areas acquired buttonhole in the flat area, so it's important to select regular topography to avoid complications and unpredictable results. A thicker cap of >100 μm as used in this study might also contribute to a lesser risk of perforation.

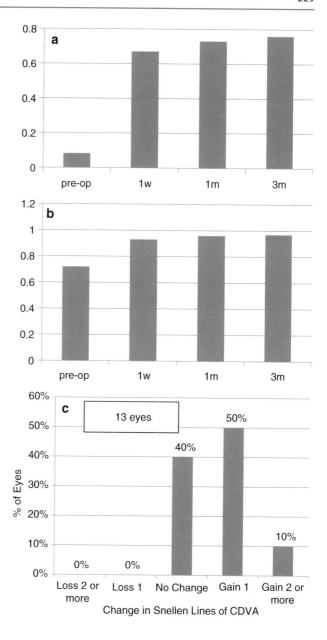

Fig. 21.9 (**a**) Mean UCVA over the follow-up period. (**b**) Mean CDVA over the follow-up period. (**c**) Safety parameters as a function of lost and gained visual acuity lines

In conclusion, SMILE procedure for the correction of post-keratoplasty myopia and astigmatism is a reproducible procedure with acceptable to good visual outcomes considering the severity of ametropia and astigmatism, in particular in these altered corneas. However, the parameters have to be modified and adjusted to the graft size. Irregular corneas should be avoided.

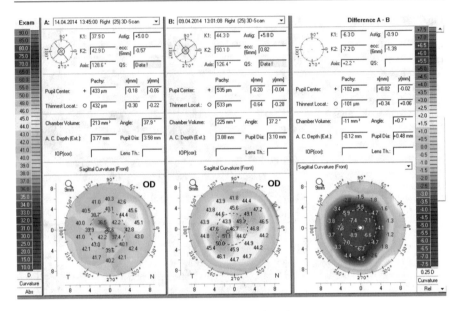

Fig. 21.10   Differential topography map of an uncomplicated case

References

1. Dan Z, Timothy J, Marine Gobbel (2014) Small incision lenticule extraction (SMILE) history, fundamentals of a new refractive surgery technique and clinical outcomes. Reinstein et al. Eye and Vision 1:3. http://www.eandv.org/content/1/1/3
2. Mastropaqua L et al (2014) Evaluation of corneal biomechanical properties. Bio Med Res Int Article ID 290619, 8 pages. http://dx.doi.org/10.1155/2014/290619
3. Reinstein DZ, Roberts C (2006) Biomechanics of corneal refractive surgery. J Refract Surg 22:285
4. Schmack I, Dawson DG, McCarey BE et al (2005) Cohesive tensile strength of human LASIK wounds with histologic, ultrastructural, and clinical correlations. J Refract Surg 21:433–445
5. Randleman JB, Dawson DG, Grossniklaus HE et al (2008) Depth-dependent cohesive tensile strength in human donor corneas: implications for refractive surgery. J Refract Surg 24: 85–89
6. Troutman RC, Gaster RN (1980) Surgical advances and results of keratoconus. Am J Ophthalmol 90:131–136
7. Azar DT, Chang JH, Han KY (2012) Wound healing after keratorefractive surgery: review of biological and optical considerations. Cornea 31(suppl 1):S9–S19
8. Güell JL, Velasco F, Roberts C et al (2005) Corneal flap thickness and topography changes induced by flap creation during laser in situ keratomileusis. J Cataract Refract Surg 31:15–119
9. Pallikaris IG, Kymionis GD, Panagopoulou SI et al (2001) Induced optical aberrations following formation of a laser in situ keratomileusis flap. J Cataract Refract Surg 28:1737–1741
10. Binder PS (2003) Ectasia after laser in situ keratomileusis. J Cataract Refract Surg 29:2419–2429

11. Wei S, Wang Y (2013) Comparison of corneal sensitivity between FS-LASIK and femtosecond lenticule extraction (ReLEx flex) or small-incision lenticule extraction (ReLEx smile) for myopic eyes. Graefes Arch Clin Exp Ophthalmol 251:1645–1654

12. Sekundo W, Kunert KS, Blum M (2011) Small incision corneal refractive surgery using the small incision lenticule extraction (SMILE) procedure for the correction of myopia and myopic astigmatism: results of a 6 month prospective study. Br J Ophthalmol 95:335–339

13. Shah R, Shah S, Sengupta S (2011) Results of small incision lenticule extraction: all-in-one femtosecond laser refractive surgery. J Cataract Refract Surg 37:127–137

14. Vestergaard A1, Ivarsen AR, Asp S, Hjortdal JØ (2012) Small-incision lenticule extraction for moderate to high myopia: Predictability, safety, and patient satisfaction. J Cataract Refract Surg. 38(11):2003–2010. doi:10.1016/j.jcrs.2012.07.021. Epub 2012 Sep 14

15. Waring GO 3rd (2000) Standard graphs for reporting refractive surgery. J Refract Surg 16:459–466

16. Reinstein DZ, Waring GO III (2009) Graphic reporting of outcomes of refractive surgery [editorial]. J Refract Surg 25:975–978

17. Dupps WJ Jr, Kohnen T, Mamalis N, Rosen ES, Koch DD, Obstbaum SA (2011) Standardized graphs and terms for refractive surgery results. J Cataract Refract Surg 37:1–3

18. Kymionis GD, Kontadakis GA, Kounis GA et al (2009) Simultaneous topography guided PRK followed by corneal collagen cross-linkage for keratoconus. J Refract Surg 25(9):807

19. Kanellopoulos AJ Short and long-term complications of combined topography guided PRK and CKL (the Athens Protocol) in 412 keratoconus eyes (22–7 years follow-up). http://laservision.gr/wp-content/uploads/2012/CKLcompsEposter-AAO11.pdf

20. Kankarriya V, Kymionis G, Kontadakis G, Yoo S (2012) Update on simultaneous topo-guided photorefractive keratoconus immediately followed by corneal collagen cross-linkage for treatment of progressive keratoconus. Int J Keratoconus Ectatic Corneal Diseases 1:185–189

Part V

Marketing and Patient Communication

How to Promote SMILE Procedure

22

Jean-François Faure and Bertram Meyer

Contents

In a context of increased competition in the refractive surgery market, surgeons who are performing SMILE have to be well prepared. They have to face overinformed patients. This chapter is written to help surgeons in their daily SMILE surgery practice. The goal is to give them keys to succeed in good marketing strategy of the all-femtosecond refractive surgery.

SMILE is a 100 % femtosecond refractive treatment with no flap; it is a single-step procedure. The femtosecond laser is used to curve the cornea.

J.-F. Faure (✉)
Espace Nouvelle Vision, Center of Refractive Surgery, Paris, France
e-mail: jf.faure@espace-nouvelle-vision.com

B. Meyer
Eye Center (Augencentrum) Cologne, Josefstraße 14, Cologne, 51143, Koeln, Germany
e-mail: Bertram.Meyer@t-online.de

© Springer International Publishing Switzerland 2015
W. Sekundo (ed.), *Small Incision Lenticule Extraction (SMILE):*
Principles, Techniques, Complication Management, and Future Concepts,
DOI 10.1007/978-3-319-18530-9_22

Promoting the new laser technology with three keywords:

Bladeless
Flapless
All-femtosecond laser procedure

22.1   Tools for Patient Recruitment

Many differences exist between the countries in terms of medical advertising. Before setting up the communication of the clinic, it is essential to take care of the legal obligations existing in connection with the promotion and to contact the public authorities. It is necessary to be sure that the way of delivering the information about the SMILE matches with the legislation in the country of your practice.

Refractive surgeons have the ethical obligation to provide accurate and truthful informative advertising. When the direct advertising is a source of conflict or unlawfulness, there are other materials and ways that can be used. Several tools are identified to help refractive surgery centers to arouse interest for SMILE among potential patients.

22.1.1 In Your Center

Create brand awareness about the superior technology available in your premium center.

1. *Leaflet*

    Brochures can be accessible for patients in refractive surgery centers or distributed during seminars. Several subtopics can be contained as the SMILE technique details and advantages, surgeons and staff qualifications. They can be a good support to diffuse the information relative to the femtosecond laser, surgical equipment, and all the preoperative technical devices which compose the refractive center equipment.

    Key point: Leaflet underlines the equipment and the staff qualities.

2. *Video support*

    They can include short clips explaining the surgery technique and advantages, but also testimonies of patients who had chosen the SMILE technique. These short informative videos can be broadcasted on video screens located in the waiting room but also on large public websites (e.g., YouTube).

    Key point: Video clips are easy to combine with the web information diffusion.

3. *The waiting room*

    The waiting room has to match with the "new technology" spirit. The design and the furnishing must be modern. Videos or brochures shorten the patient waiting time and can give desire for people or patients who come for classical consultation to learn more about SMILE surgery.

Key point: The waiting room is the refractive center's showroom and always a source of potential refractive patients.

4. *Qualified staff*

Surgeons have to remember that they are their best advertising. Patients are very attentive to the image reflected by their surgeon's personality, but also by the image of his staff. They have to be as qualified as much as possible and be aware of the refractive surgery methods which exist, including SMILE. It will give a positive image of the staff, the clinic, and the practice. All of them are representatives of the seriousness and quality of the patient's care provided.

Key point: Refractive center staff members and surgeons behaviors are the best advertising for SMILE technique.

22.1.2 Outside of Your Center

Involve everybody with campaigns to spread the message and incentives for performing higher numbers at all levels.

The campaigns must be especially targeting the youth.

1. *Website*

SMILE is a refractive surgery technique available for all myopic patients. The patient's profile corresponds to people who are well informed about new technologies. They are on demand for the state-of-the-art surgery technique. These patients can be easily recruited using the Internet marketing. The investment in a website showing your clinic, your practice, and your prices is certainly cost effective. The correct presentation of the surgeon to whom the potential refractive candidate is going to entrust his vision is of particular importance (Figs. 22.1, 22.2). The SMILE technique can be easily detailed with some illustrative animations or figures. A section providing answers to the frequently asked questions can be inserted. If the website is run by a qualified staff, it can also include a section where people can ask their own questions and communicate by e-mail. A section to schedule the first check makes it easy for most of them if they want to go further. To guarantee a regular updating and the long-term website viability, a section with scientific papers about the SMILE can be created. The website can also provide to patients a forum to share their experience before and after the surgery. To avoid negative communication, this forum must stay under the control of a qualified administrator. To optimize the website, it seems relevant to invest on advertising campaign for better search engine results (= SEO). The semantic integration can also improve the natural referencing. This last part in managing the website can be delegated to a specialized company which certainly prevents a waste of time and money.

Key point: A website well matches with the SMILE potential patient's profile.

2. *Social networks (e.g., Facebook, Xing, Google+, etc.)*

Ask patients for interactivities and positive comments in social network platforms and "refractive" chatrooms. Encourage them to share their positive

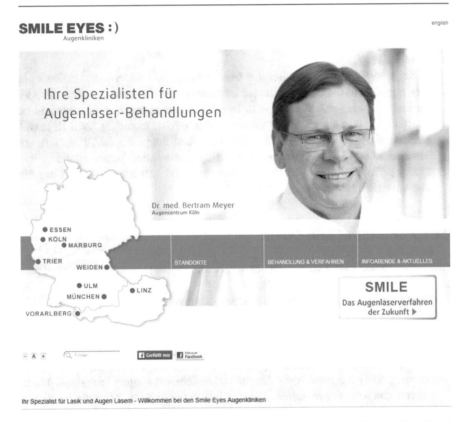

Fig. 22.1 An example of the presenting website of one of the authors. According to a "local hero" principle, the surgeon is presented first. Two other points are emphasized at the same time *without overloading* the front page: Your surgeon is a true specialist in LVC who, of course, offers the advanced procedure "SMILE." All other detailed information are given when the potential customer clicks on other buttons

experiences with others and to recommend the positive atmosphere in your clinic prior, during, and after SMILE surgery. Positive and emotional comments are repressing fears and scares.

3. *Traditional print media, radio, and TV*

You can set up editorials or advertorials in daily newspapers or lifestyle magazines (including aviation, railway magazines, etc.) and smart and "sexy" spots on TV and radio. But be aware that all these activities are very expensive, have a lot of dead loss, and are also giving indirect benefit to your competitors. Last but not least, please note that the "young laser generation" which we want to catch is more focused on the Internet than on traditional media

4. *Create, manage, and develop a network of SMILE experts*

This network is composed by all the health professionals who are likely to refer patients for refractive surgery. Of course, other ophthalmologists who do not

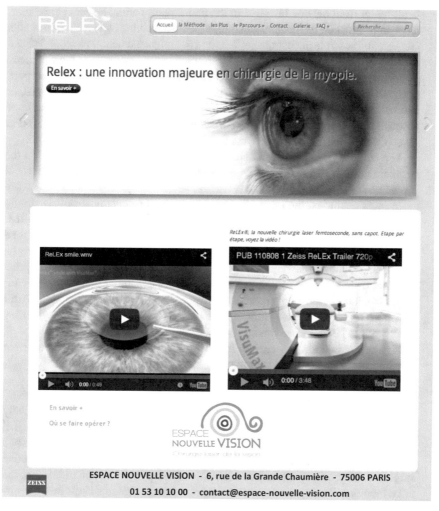

Fig. 22.2 This website is dedicated to the SMILE technique, focusing on the future patient expectations. They can watch short videos presenting the laser technology

practice refractive surgery are part of it, but also the opticians and optometrists in the neighborhood and the general practitioners. As they are health-care professionals, they represent a good way to spread information. Patients feel in a trustworthy relationship, because they have no financial interest to refer them. Unlike the surgeons, they benefit from an image of proximity. Their opinions and advices are more often sought for and listened to. By referring a patient, they are at the beginning of the surgery process and the patient feels well surrounded. Depending on the relationship which already exists, a member of the staff clinic can visit these health professionals to introduce them to the SMILE surgery. The message needs to be complete, accurate, and easy to understand. The information delivered must be different from the one intended to the mainstream public. It seems to be more relevant to insist on technical details, postoperative results, patient's comfort after surgery, and possible undesirable effects and their management. In a second phase, the referrals have to be integrated to the refractive care pathway of their patients. The clinic must consider them as partners to maintain good relationship. The postoperative report can be sent, and in the particular case of other ophthalmologist, he can be in charge of the postoperative follow-up. To maintain the connection, a newsletter treating of SMILE press review can be sent every month by e-mail or letter. Occasionally, the refractive center can organize a meeting on that issue.

Key point: Referral network consists in an effective information relay. At the beginning of this eye care pathway, they have to be considered as partners.

5. *Phone calls*

In most countries, the telemarketing is perceived as unethical or it is simply illegal. But thanks to the other ways of communication, potential ReLEx SMILE patients can call for further information. People who answer the phone must be well informed about the refractive surgery SMILE technique. They have to be able to answer most questions. Otherwise, interested people could get the impression that the SMILE technique is far from tight. Remember that new technologies, especially in the medical field, are frightening to most of the patients. After refractive surgery, they just want to have perfect vision without glasses but they don't want to be part of a clinical trial.

Key point: Phone calls consist in direct advertising with telemarketing but also indirect as an additional support to other ways of communication.

6. *Price policy*

Prices are difficult to transfer with respect to ethical consideration and legislation. As it is common in the refractive surgery market, the demand is relatively highly correlated with price: as price comes down, demand goes up. The SMILE must be associated with the state-of-the-art refractive surgery concept. It is not a low-cost surgery. Concerning the price positioning among the other refractive surgery techniques, it has to be at the top of the pyramid. Remember that the price includes the surgeon fees which represent the surgeon's skills and the surgical tools and equipment used. PRK or LASIK cost must be cheaper than SMILE procedures.

Key point: As SMILE is the most sophisticated refractive surgery technique, it must be the most expensive one.

7. *Vouchers and incentives*

If patients are recommending your clinic straight ahead to friends and family or others and if those recommendations are directly resulting in a refractive procedure (esp. SMILE), you can give – as a kind of appreciation – a "financial voucher" to the recommending person and/or a small discount to ongoing patients. Nevertheless, this way of marketing is not always easy to handle and requires sensitivity and tact.

8. *The word from mouth to ear*

This is one of the last but most important ways to attract potential patients for the SMILE surgery. Patients talk about SMILE with their social environment. When they are satisfied with the refractive and visual outcome, this will have extraordinary positive consequences on your activity. The practice of SMILE surgery on famous and well-known people or persons of influence is less costly but really effective. During postoperative care surgeons can ask them to share their experience with others and – why not – realize short video clips or publish their testimonies online. These people are considered as those who are always going one step ahead. If they have chosen SMILE technique, it must be the best one for refractive correction, on the cutting edge of technology.

Key point: The word from mouth to ear has to be encouraged among patients who already have undergone SMILE.

22.2   Tools to Convert the Refractive Candidates into SMILE Refractive Patients

Converting all LASIK patients to SMILE

Up-to-date patients prefer premium services and more advanced surgical techniques which offer superior outcomes.

Believe in the technology to make it work for you.

First case: The patient doesn't know anything about refractive surgery procedure. Talk to him directly about SMILE; it is not necessary to convert and speak about any other procedure than LASIK or PRK.

Second case: The patient knows the LASIK or PRK procedure but nothing about SMILE. Speak to him to convert with evidence.

Third case: The patient has heard about SMILE and wants this procedure. It is easy to expose the benefit of this treatment. You must ask him which ways allowed him to discover this method. Knowing these ways can give you directions to develop your own communication.

Several tools can help surgeons to convert SMILE interest into SMILE surgery among potential refractive patients. This second part on the patient's pathway provides a non-exhaustive list of the key arguments supporting SMILE technique and helping surgeons to be persuasive.

22.2.1 Discussion with the Future Patients

In order to convince patients of the benefits of SMILE surgery, the surgeon has to take time for his explanations. The information transferred has to be patient oriented and to be communicated in simple words. During the discussion, explicative supports as brochures can help. The SMILE surgery must be introduced to the patient as an established refractive treatment, offering a maximum of protection for a minimum of constraints.

The future of laser vision correction is:

100 % bladeless
100 % flapless
100 % all-femtosecond laser procedure

1. *The equipment qualities*

It is as important as taking a flight. Passengers have to trust in their pilot's skills and in aircraft's technology.

To be convinced, a patient must be in good terms with his future surgeon, but he also has to trust in the surgical facilities.

The surgeon has to create a confidential climate and underline the advantages and qualities of the technical devices he is using to succeed in SMILE surgery.

SMILE represents the state-of-the-art refractive surgery technique. It seems more convenient to use surgical disposable products for this refractive surgery, which allows a better peroperative safety.

2. *The femtosecond laser*

There is only one laser in the refractive market worldwide which allows to perform SMILE procedure. The laser VisuMax® (Carl Zeiss Meditec AG) provides numerous benefits: predictability, efficacy, stability, and precision. The success of the SMILE surgery and the excellent visual outcomes obtained are partly due to this equipment's qualities. It represents the latest state-of-the-art femtosecond surgery which is now the third generation in laser refractive surgery. The advantages offered by this femtosecond laser can be easily identified and understood by the potential patients.

3. *Minimal incision size*

The femtosecond laser allows a minimally invasive procedure with less than a 2.5 mm incision. As a direct consequence, this provides a greater corneal integrity. The upper layer of the cornea remains mainly intact and this preserves corneal biomechanical stability, offering a maximum of protection.

4. *Less ocular dryness after surgery*

During the postoperative days, the patient comfort is improved compared to other surgical techniques because of minimal reaction in the cornea. The upper layer remains untouched and the corneal nerve section is cut only less than 2.5 mm. The corneal nerves are partly responsible for the lacrimal secretion. As the SMILE preserves these corneal nerves, the lacrimal secretion is less disturbed and the postoperative dryness is reduced. It must be underlined that SMILE causes less severe dry eye syndrome.

5. *Single-step procedure*

The all-femtosecond refractive surgery is a single-step procedure, with no need to move the patient to another bed. This reduces his stress situation.

6. *Flapless*

It is a flapless procedure which means for patient that there is no risk to lose vision quality after surgery because of a flap accident.

To lift and to re-put a human tissue is not without consequence, during and after the surgery. With SMILE, the access for germs or bacteria to the interface is tremendously reduced. Moreover, no flap lift means no organic flap complications (e.g., microstriae, folds, dislocation, etc.)

7. *Rapid laser action*

The creation of the lenticule during the SMILE surgery is one of the shortest procedures. To the patient's side, it is reassuring to know that just the laser surgery will not last more than 25 s.

8. *Comfortable equipment*

The patient's comfort during surgery must also be considered as an advantage. He is lying on a bed with an intelligent head. Monitoring the patient's position and minimal movements, the system will automatically adjust during the treatment.

9. *Natural design of the contact glass*

The design of the contact glass is made to fit with the anatomy of the ocular surface. The curved shape of the contact glass, similar to the cornea's shape, avoids vision complications caused by a twist of the cutting plan during the three-dimensional curved lenticule's creation.

10. *Soft corneal suction*

Compared to other refractive lasers, the real corneal suction time is short and without discomfort for the patient. The effective suction on the patient's eye starts 4 s prior to the lenticule's creation. The pressure on the eye is much less compared to other lasers, but it is strong enough to keep the eye positioned during the treatment. This avoids intraocular pressure complications.

11. *Safety assets and permanent surgeon control*

The surgical microscope equipped with digital video camera gives the surgeon a visual control during the entire procedure for a maximum of safety. The femtosecond precision associated to the high-precision optics provides an extremely focused laser beam. The result is a high level of accuracy, predictability and an extremely precise visual outcomes.

12. *Noiseless and odorless*

Compared to the other procedure, the VisuMax allows a noiseless and odorless surgery which is much less uncomfortable and disturbing for patients.

13. *Preoperative technical devices*

The quality of the topographer and wavefront analyzer guarantees the precision of the measurements taken prior to surgery.

14. *Quick vision recovery*

The vision recovery after a SMILE is almost the same as in LASIK and much faster than a PRK. After a few days, nearly all patients have full preoperative visual acuity.

15. *Quick way back to sports*

As it is a flapless and less invasive procedure, patients can return to sports practice almost immediately after the surgery. The risk of complication due to potential mechanical shock or bacterial invasion (for swimmers) is close to zero.

16. *Real alternative to PRK*

Patients' way of life or profession sometimes prohibits LASIK surgery. Before SMILE was established on the market, the only solution for flapless visual and refractive rehabilitation was PRK, but it is causing days of inability to work or to practice sports. Military people, firefighters, policemen, and persons doing contact sports have now an excellent alternative. SMILE is the surgery of reference especially for them.

17. *Patient can put on "makeup" shortly after surgery*

With less than 2,5 mm incision, there is no contraindication to restart makeup the day after surgery.

18. *No need of protective hard covers*

The all-femtosecond refractive surgery causes corneal biomechanical stress at its minimum. As it is a flapless procedure, there is no need to wear protection shields in order to avoid mechanical complication.

SMILE does not only revolutionize the technological part of the refractive surgery market but also patients' postoperative way of life. After SMILE, they can immediately return to their daily activity with nearly no risk of complications. SMILE represents a minimum of constraints and gives a maximum of postoperative comfort.

22.3 Eventual Adverse Events

A good marketing in refractive surgery does not only consist in listing all the advantages but also to talk about the eventual adverse events and the way to manage it. Patient will feel safer, if their surgeon knows how to proceed when facing difficulties. With the SMILE technique, there are few peroperative and postoperative adverse events easy to manage with no consequence on long-term visual outcomes postoperatively. It seems important to communicate to patients that even if SMILE is the most sophisticated refractive surgery technique, there is never zero risk.

22.3.1 Peroperative Adverse Events

The three main peroperative adverse events are very rare and do not cause loss of vision after refractive surgery failure.

22.3.1.1 Suction Loss

During the femtosecond step, a contact glass fixes the patient's eye with a gentle pressure. In 0.75 % of cases, the suction is released before the end of the complete lenticule's creation. Depending on the time when the suction is released, the SMILE procedure can be restarted. In very rare cases, it is not possible and the procedure could not be completed. In these cases the patient will easily understand that it is safer to reschedule a new surgery using a PRK or LASIK procedure.

22.3.1.2 Dissection in the Wrong Layer

The plan dissection difficulties concern 0.6 % of the lenticule's preparation. For the patient's side it could be uncomfortable because it increases the surgery time only. The surgeon has to process more tricky and slowly.

22.3.1.3 Secondary Fracture Line Close to the Incision

This may happen due to a lot of mechanical strength or a patient's eye movement during preparation. This occurs in less than 0.3 % of all preparations. It does not require a special management, just a classical follow-up by checking the complete healing.

22.3.2 Common Postoperative Adverse Events

The recovery period usually lasts 4–5 h. Some patients have the experience of an extended time of blurred vision or dry eye or increased light sensitivity. These adverse events are common to LASIK and SMILE surgery, are unpredictable, and depend on individual patient characteristics.

As all the postoperative adverse events, they are a source of postoperative discomfort for patients, but they are temporary and do not cause visual loss or corneal damages on long term.

22.3.3 Epithelial Cells Remaining on the Interface

Usually not on the visual axis, some epithelial cells can remain in the interface and potentially grow. If the vision is disturbed, a simple procedure of Nd:YAG or a washout with a simple irrigation of the interface will be enough to remove those cells. It happens in 0.6 % of the lenticule's extractions.

22.4 Classical Mistakes in the SMILE Marketing

All the refractive surgeons who practice or will practice the SMILE have the obligation to transfer a good branding of this technique. To be convincing and to contribute to the development of the SMILE technique, they have to be aware about the classical mistakes made to avoid them during their explanations to the patients:

1. Confusing the surgeon's attempts with those of the patients

   The real desire of patients is to have a surgeon with highest qualifications and with best clinical results.

   When the SMILE technique is introduced, the two first reasons to convince are the excellent visual outcomes and the safety of this procedure. The technological proofs are only used in a second time. During the explanations it is important to insist on the overall future experience for the patient and not only to focus on the clinical advantages.

2. The clinical trial image

After surgery patients just want to see clearly without risk. SMILE must not be presented as a new concept; it is just a new way to proceed surgery with a new refractive tool. The concept is not recent. Reshaping the cornea to give patient visual rehabilitation without glasses or contact lenses is the same as for all the corneal refractive techniques. More than 25 years of experience in the refractive laser surgery contributes to set up the small incision lenticule extraction.

3. Introducing SMILE as a niche market

SMILE is not a surgical technique available only for patients who have spherical myopia or to those who usually have up-to-date technological preoccupations. It is the reference treatment in laser refractive surgery accessible for myopia from −1.00 to −10.00 diopters and astigmatism up to −5 diopters. The correction of hyperopia and presbyopia is expected on the market in the near future.

4. Bashing LASIK or PRK procedure

Even if the SMILE is the state-of-the-art refractive surgery technique, LASIK or PRK will still be a good refractive technique. There are about 25 years of good clinical results which provide information and experience to create and develop the SMILE.

Key point: Do not alarm patients with this new SMILE procedure. Communicate that it is not a new technique but the use of a more accurate, more predictable, and safer laser only. Point out that all myopia patients treated in your hands benefit from the SMILE procedure now.

Conclusion

In the next few years, SMILE will definitively rise to the most dominant refractive procedure performed. Only good refractive surgeons will be able to practice SMILE. Both their technical skills and their marketing strategy will make the difference.

Erratum

Small Incision Lenticule Extraction (SMILE)

Walter Sekundo, Editor

ISBN 978-3-319-18529-3

Erratum to:

Book ESMs and few chapter ESMs have been included in the Springer link. The copyright page holds the video link and the cover contains "Extras online" logo.

The video link included in the copyright page is:

http://springerextras.com/978-3-319-18529-3

© Springer International Publishing Switzerland 2015
W. Sekundo (ed.), *Small Incision Lenticule Extraction (SMILE):
Principles, Techniques, Complication Management, and Future Concepts,*
DOI 10.1007/978-3-319-18530-9_23

Printed in the United States
By Bookmasters